MEDICAL PRACTICE

Body of Knowledge Review

VOLUME 7

Planning and Marketing

Reid M. Oetjen, PhD, MSHSA

Dawn M. Oetjen, PhD, MHA

Managing Editor
Lawrence F. Wolper, MBA, FACMPE

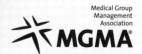

Medical Group
Management
Association

Medical Group Management Association
104 Inverness Terrace East
Englewood, CO 80112-5306
877.275.6462
Website: www.mgma.com

Medical Group Management Association (MGMA) publications are intended to provide current and accurate information and are designed to assist readers in becoming more familiar with the subject matter covered. Such publications are distributed with the understanding that MGMA does not render any legal, accounting, or other professional advice that may be construed as specifically applicable to an individual situation. No representations or warranties are made concerning the application of legal or other principles discussed by the authors to any specific factual situation, nor is any prediction made concerning how any particular judge, government official, or other person will interpret or apply such principles. Specific factual situations should be discussed with professional advisors.

Production Credits
Executive Editor: Andrea M. Rossiter, FACMPE
Managing Editor: Lawrence F. Wolper, MBA, FACMPE
Editorial Director: Marilee E. Aust
Production Editor: Marti A. Cox, MLIS
Substantive and Copy Editor: Sandra Rush, Rush Services
Proofreaders: Scott Vickers, InstEdit and Karen Krizman
Page Design, Composition and Production: Boulder Bookworks
Cover Design: Ian Serff, Serff Creative Group, Inc.

PUBLISHER'S CATALOGING IN PUBLICATION DATA

Oetjen, Reid M.
 Planning and marketing / by Reid M. Oetjen, Dawn M. Oetjen ; managing editor Lawrence F. Wolper. – Englewood, CO : MGMA, 2006.
 146 p. : 5 ill. ; cm. – (Medical Practice Management Body of Knowledge Review Series ; v. 7)
Includes index.
ISBN 1-56829-237-6
 1. Group medical practice—Marketing. [LC] 2. Marketing of health services. [MeSH] 3. Business planning. [LC] 4. Strategic planning [LC] I. Oetjen, Dawn M. II. Wolper, Lawrence F. III. Medical Group Management Association. IV. American College of Medical Practice Executives. V. Series. VI. Series: Body of Knowledge Review Series.

R728.O38 2006
610.68.O38—dc22   2005938858

Item 6358

ISBN: 1-56829-237-6   Library of Congress Control Number: 2005938858

Printed in the United States of America
10 9 8 7 6 5 4 3 2 1

Contents

Series Overview

THE MEDICAL GROUP MANAGEMENT ASSOCIATION (MGMA) serves medical practices of all sizes, as well as management services organizations, integrated delivery systems, and ambulatory surgery centers to assist members with information, education, networking, and advocacy. Through the American College of Medical Practice Executives® (ACMPE®), MGMA's standard-setting and certification body, the organization provides board certification and Fellowship in medical practice management and supports those seeking to advance their careers.

■ **Core Learning Series: A professional development pathway for competency and excellence in medical practice management**

Medical practice management is one of the fastest-growing and most rewarding careers in health care administration. It is also one of the most demanding, requiring a breadth of skills and knowledge unique to the group practice environment. For these reasons, MGMA and ACMPE have created a comprehensive series of learning resources, customized to meet the specific professional development needs of medical practice managers: the *Medical Practice Management Core Learning Series*.

The Medical Practice Management Core Learning Series is a structured approach that enables practice administrators and staff to build the core knowledge and skills required for career success. Series resources include seminars, Web-based education programs, books, and online assessment tools. These resources provide a strong, expansive foundation for managing myriad job responsibilities and daily challenges.

■ Core Learning Series: Resources for understanding medical practice operations

To gain a firm footing in medical practice management, executives need a broad understanding of the knowledge and skills required to do the job. The Medical Practice Management Core Learning Series offers "Level 1" resources, which provide an introduction to the essentials of medical practice management. As part of the learning process, professionals can use these resources to assess their current level of knowledge across all competency areas, identify gaps in their education or experience, and select areas in which to focus further study. The *Medical Practice Management Body of Knowledge Review Series* is considered to be a Core Learning Series – Level 1 resource.

Level 1 resources meet the professional development needs of individuals who are new to or considering a career in the field of medical practice management, assuming practice management responsibilities, or considering ACMPE board certification in medical practice management.

Also offered are Core Learning Series – Level 2 resources, which provide exposure to more advanced concepts in specific competency areas and their application to day-to-day operation of the medical practice. These resources meet the needs of individuals who have more experience in the field, who seek specialized knowledge in a particular area of medical practice management, and/or who are completing preparations for the ACMPE board certification examinations.

■ Core Learning Series: Resources to become board certified

Board certification and Fellowship in ACMPE are well-earned badges of professional achievement. The designations Certified Medical Practice Executive (CMPE) and Fellow in ACMPE (FACMPE) indicate that the professional has attained significant levels of expertise across the full range of the medical practice administrator's responsibilities. The Medical Practice Management Core Learning Series is MGMA's recommended learning system for certification preparation. With attainment of the CMPE designation, practice executives will be well positioned to excel in their careers through ACMPE Fellowship.

Preface

TODAY'S MEDICAL GROUP PRACTICES are continually faced with change – change in reimbursement; change in financial and organizational oversight; change in leadership; and change in policies, regulations, and standards; as well as change in the health care needs and wants of the populations served.

To survive this hyperturbulent and complex change of pace in health care, medical practice executives must be adaptable. Strategic planning allows the practice to change direction in a quick and consistent fashion. Strategic planning is a powerful tool that can help medical group practices achieve goals and objectives on a continuous basis, especially as they relate to a rapidly changing, dynamic environment.[1] Successful medical practice executives will be those who embrace strategic planning and marketing, rather than those who are merely reactive to their environments. Despite this need, the majority of medical group practices have not participated in strategic planning.

The strategic plan can serve as a powerful foundation on which to base a more detailed and comprehensive business plan. A business plan precisely defines the practice, identifies its goals, and serves as its operational resume. An effective business plan can help medical practices to allocate resources effectively and facilitate sound business decision making. This book provides medical practice executives with a means to develop effective plans to aid in decision making.

Additionally, the growth of consumerism and the technological changes in the delivery of health care pose challenges to medical groups. Medical practice executives will be exposed to an arsenal of marketing tools to take advantage of these opportunities. An effective marketing plan incorporates much of the information of the strategic and business plans, but shifts the focus to the external environment. At the strategic level, marketing should be directed at scanning the environment, predicting what is happening, and looking for emerging trends or robust market segments to target.

It is not enough to simply develop strategic, business, and marketing plans; rather, medical practice executives must continually monitor and evaluate the planning activities and the status of implementation of the plan. Practice executives will learn a systematic method for measuring the effectiveness of these plans, which must be established so that clear links between past, present, and future strategies and results can be determined. Additionally, monitoring and evaluation can help medical practice executives to extract relevant information from past and ongoing activities that can subsequently be used for fine-tuning strategies. Without a formal process for monitoring and evaluation, it would be impossible to assess the effectiveness of current strategies and to improve future efforts.

To survive in today's turbulent health care market, it is essential that organizations position themselves by forming strategic alliances. Alliances are not new to health care; they have been a part of the medical practice landscape for years. The success of a medical group often rests with the practice executive's ability to forge alliances in which diverse individuals and interests collaborate and leverage resources. In this volume, medical practice executives will be introduced to the different forms of alliances and how to approach the formation of these strategic partnerships.

Furthermore, to prosper in today's health care market, a group practice must employ a long-term strategy that is driven by commitment, continuity, and consistency so that its relationship with the community can be sustained.[2] Medical practice managers must build trust and commitment within the community and among the customers they serve. To do so, medical practices need to become actively engaged in the community in which they operate. An effective method to accomplish this is to develop programs aimed at the community.

The objective of this volume is to provide insight for medical practice executives into the strategic planning and marketing process. Medical practice executives must have a vision of the past, present, and – most important – the future, and must succeed in communicating such a vision to others in a way that their followers adopt the vision as their own. This volume presents concepts of strategic planning and marketing based on sound business practice tailored to the medical practice environment. The intent is for practice executives to use the tools and knowledge provided to better manage their organizations and resources.

Learning Objectives

AFTER READING THIS VOLUME, the medical practice executive will be able to:

1. Analyze and interpret market research data to help guide strategic planning for the practice;

2. Communicate business-planning factors to physicians and staff to influence movement in synchronization with emerging trends;

3. Generate ideas to target markets and meet the needs of diverse demographic segments;

4. Organize public, customer, and community relations programs to communicate the key messages and image of the practice;

5. Evaluate promotion methods to maximize "best fit" for each market segment;

6. Assess needs for additional ancillary services that fit with the practice's mission and vision;

7. Negotiate external affiliations for the practice;

8. Serve as a role model for effectively dealing with stress and ambiguity to help physicians and staff cope with change;

9. Negotiate legal and financial contracts with marketing vendors to ensure the best cost/benefit ratio for practice resources;

10. Facilitate ongoing monitoring of business and marketing plans and make appropriate adjustments in line with medical industry dynamics;

11. Build consensus on the most appropriate marketing mix to complement the strategic plan; and

12. Design new products/services to foster practice growth and better serve customers.

How Outreach Can Strengthen Your Practice

MEDICAL PRACTICES invested in community service have found unexpected returns for their businesses. Those benefits range from kinder treatment from payers to exceptional patient opinions to physician loyalty. Call it smart business, or call it good karma, but what goes around does come around.

Consider, for example, the clinicians of Bluegrass Orthopaedics in Lexington, Ky. They spend about 20 hours a month at local health fairs providing free screenings for osteoporosis. They use the practice's $37,000 mobile heel scanner, purchased six years ago, for just that purpose.

"When I started with this practice in 1996, the three founding physicians felt very deeply about heading in this direction," says MGMA member and Bluegrass practice administrator Cynthia L. Dunn, FACMPE. "We have the responsibility to give back to our community and in particular to educate people about osteoporosis because it is so preventable."

The practice also participates in school scoliosis screenings (to detect spinal curvature), airport ergonomics seminars, and wellness luncheon speeches at hospitals – all done free of charge as part of the eight-physician practice's mission to improve community health.

However, Dunn is acutely aware of the health care axiom, "no margin, no mission." Bluegrass Orthopaedics competes with not one but two dominant players – the orthopedic departments of the University of Kentucky and Lexington Clinic. And so, community service not only has star billing in the practice's mission, it also plays a supporting role in its business plan to build Bluegrass Orthopaedics' name recognition.

"Participating in our community and becoming known in it is no doubt helpful to our marketing," Dunn says.

■ Charity Begins at Home

Reaching out to the community can bolster the business side of a practice in three ways, says Sandra W. Reifsteck, RN, MS, FACMPE, MGMA member, and Great Plains regional consultant, Institute for Healthcare Communication, New Haven, Conn. The exposure can attract new patients, strengthen the loyalty of current patients, and fortify a practice's long-range planning. "Practices that want to be strong, progressive businesses in their markets must develop clear visions of the future. And that means they have to be involved in their communities," says Reifsteck, the former associate administrator of outreach and development with Carle Clinic Association, Urbana, Ill., for 25 years.

Reifsteck was the founder of the Carle Community Parish Nurse Program, Carle Clinic Association & Carle Foundation Hospital in Urbana, Ill., the 2003 recipient of the ACMPE-MGMA Fred Graham Award for Innovation in Improving Community Health. The award recognizes practices' innovative solutions to advance the effectiveness of health care delivery and improve community health. Since 1997, the Carle Community Parish Nurse Program has trained parish nurses to provide a range of services to their community, including assistance to families, support for family transitions, and bereavement counseling. "We felt we could make the most lasting impact by getting into churches because then we really were out in the community," Reifsteck says.

Any medical practice probably has a pile of community service possibilities. All that is needed is a leadership spark for them to catch fire. Reifsteck recommends that medical practice executives take a close look at their own practices and ask these three questions:

   ■ What are the practice's talents, and interests?

- What does the practice's mission say?
- Where is the "low-hanging fruit" – what do data show about the needs in the community?

"Be sure you've clearly thought out the reasons to do community service. Physicians are busy, and you have to give them reasons to do this," Reifsteck says. She also advises practices to start small and look for ways to collaborate, for example by participating in a program already offered by payers or hospitals.

"Partnerships are key. You have the expertise, while others in the community may have the resources. Most physicians' offices can only do so much," Reifsteck says.

■ Keeping Patient Populations Healthy

The 2004 recipient of the Fred Graham Award, Women's Healthcare Associates LLC (WHA) in Beaverton, Ore., provides prenatal services to undocumented – and thus uninsured – workers, most of whom are Hispanic. "Doing crisis medicine was no good for us or for patients, so we have a self-interest in keeping all of our patient populations healthy," says Brian P. Kelly, CMPE, MGMA member, and chief executive officer of WHA.

Each year, WHA provides services to approximately 600 pregnant undocumented workers. Thanks to WHA and its partner organization, Providence St. Vincent Hospital, Washington County statistics show that nearly 78 percent of pregnant Hispanic women there receive care in the first trimester, compared with 65 percent of Hispanic women statewide. Only 50 out of 1,000 Hispanic babies born in the county have low birth weight – the least among Hispanics and non-Hispanics within the Portland metropolitan tri-counties as well as the state. Two physicians and four certified nurse midwives from WHA give 18 hours of clinic time per week, and the hospital provides the facilities, billing, clinic support, nurses, a receptionist, a nurse practitioner, case management, and administrative assistance.

■ Giving Physicians a Reason to Stay

Just 100 miles south of WHA, in Eugene, Ore., community service is what PeaceHealth Medical Group is all about. The group is part of PeaceHealth, a not-for-profit health care system sponsored by the Sisters of St. Joseph of Peace, with services in Oregon, Washington, and Alaska.

The system's mission is to take care of anyone who walks in the door, says Chris A. Clarke, CMPE, MGMA member, and vice president of operations of PeaceHealth Medical Group. That includes the 47,000 potential new patients who used PeaceHealth's urgent care clinic last year. "We're fortunate that we've been able to ensure that we can continue the work started by the Sisters, and that includes broadening access by bringing in new patients," Clarke says.

PeaceHealth features myriad community services, including two health information libraries open to anyone in the community and free assistance from three full-time staff members devoted to helping patients apply for pharmaceutical companies' free medications. PeaceHealth measures its community image with surveys and focus groups, and the results, says Clarke, are "always very positive." Through these means, the community recently asked PeaceHealth to direct more community service to wellness and wellness education, and the organization is listening.

PeaceHealth's devotion to community service has had an unplanned benefit: easier physician recruitment and better retention among its 300 employed physicians. "When we ask physicians during their first year why they chose PeaceHealth, 99 percent say the reason is our mission," Clarke says. PeaceHealth's retention rate figures reflect that support – compared with the average physician turnover rate of 10 to 15 percent, theirs is just 4 percent.

PeaceHealth chooses projects that will "give the community the biggest benefit," says Clarke. PeaceHealth is now collaborating with other health care providers outside its system to open a federally qualified health center in Eugene/Springfield.

■ Getting Back by Giving

A record 45 million Americans – or almost one in six – lacked health care coverage in 2003. In 2002, the total was 43.6 million. The previous high was 44.3 million in 1998.[3] This comes as no surprise, as the cost of health insurance has risen 59 percent since 2000.[4]

Even doing what some physicians already believe is community service – practicing in medically underserved areas or accepting Medicaid patients (and in some areas and specialties, Medicare patients) – can have its own unexpected rewards.

"We have credibility with the health plans and hospitals because of our prenatal program. They know we don't 'cherry pick' patients," says WHA's Kelly. "And it has made our relationships smoother. One health plan, in fact, says it values practices that take on more than their share and looks harder at the practices that don't accept Medicaid. When we need problems solved with hospitals and health plans, the doors are open and it's easier."[5]

Igniting the blaze of excitement for community service is one thing; keeping it under control is quite another. Part of being a professional practice administrator is helping to set parameters for what the practice can and cannot do in its community service.

Planning and Marketing and the General Competencies

The *ACMPE Guide to the Body of Knowledge for Medical Practice Management* identifies five general competencies expected of practice executives. These five competencies demonstrate an executive's (1) Professionalism, (2) Leadership, (3) Communication skills, (4) Organizational and Analytical Skills, and (5) Technical/Professional Knowledge and Skills. Each of these competencies plays a role in carrying out the tasks in the Planning and Marketing domain.

■ Professionalism

The ACMPE *Guide* defines the Professionalism competency as "demonstrating a commitment to achieving professional standards that enhance personal and organizational integrity and contribute to the profession." An important aspect of planning is that, if done well, it creates a perception of professionalism. By planning thoroughly and developing a strategic vision supported by practical documents – in the form of strategic, business, and marketing plans – a serious commitment to the practice's future is demonstrated. From this commitment, professionalism can be inferred. A professional environment will emerge within the practice and, internally, become a part of the culture of the organization. Externally, the practice will be viewed as visionary and professional as well.

■ Leadership

According to the *Guide*, "medical practice executives must demonstrate leadership by collaborating with and supporting the practice's physician leadership to provide strategic direction to the organization and the operational systems to carry it out." This is, essentially, a statement about planning. Collaborating with the practice's internal and external stakeholders; researching and developing strategic direction in the form of mission, vision, and goals and strategies; and identifying and ensuring that the operational systems and resources needed to complete plan implementation are available are the cornerstones of planning. Leadership is the means to accomplish these tasks.

■ Communication Skills

The ACMPE *Guide* defines the Communication competency as a "demonstration of communication skills necessary to elicit multiple points of view from internal and external sources, facilitate constructive interaction, and present information clearly and concisely." Each of the plans – strategic, business, and marketing – is an exercise in communicating to stakeholders the practice's past, present, and future status. The first step in implementing these plans is to get key people to actually read them. If the intent of these plans is not clearly and concisely articulated, there is the chance they will not be read or that they will not receive the needed buy-in for success, which would render them useless. Communication skills are therefore an integral part of the planning and marketing process.

■ Organizational and Analytical Skills

The ACMPE *Guide* defines this competency as "demonstrating a systematic approach to problem solving, decision making, and the development and administration of systems to address day-to-day issues and the long-term improvement needs of the practice." The planning and marketing processes are actual demonstrations of an executive's organizational and analytical skills. Meticulously adhering to each step in the development of a plan, understanding the information required, scheduling the implementation, and then monitoring and evaluating the plan on a regular basis require excellent organizational and analytical skills. Without this competency, planning and marketing within the practice would surely falter.

■ Technical/Professional Knowledge and Skills

The fifth competency, Technical/Professional Knowledge and Skills, is the competency in which the domain of Planning and Marketing is most integral. This competency is defined by the *Guide* as a "demonstration of the knowledge and skills for competent job performance." In any health care environment, all practice executives must be able to plan – and then execute the plan successfully. This is especially critical in today's rapidly changing health care environment. Executives have to stay one step ahead of trends; they must strive to develop new strategies and keep ahead of competition as well. Planning and marketing are professional skills that, in order to be practiced, require vast knowledge of the practice – in particular, the internal and external environments. It is up to the practice executive to ensure that the practice is in a position for future success. Utilizing the executive's technical/professional knowledge and skills to assist in planning and marketing for the practice is one way to accomplish this.

Current Planning and Marketing Issues

MEDICAL PRACTICES are faced with an ever-increasing amount of social, economic, political, and competitive pressures. The pace of change in health care has become so rapid and complex that it is essential that practice executives have a firm grasp on strategic planning. Another vital skill for medical practice executives is to have an arsenal of strategic planning and marketing tools so they can take advantage of opportunities.

Medical group practices have experienced substantial changes in how they market their services due to internal organizational as well as external environmental forces. According to a recent study of 11 leading academic medical centers conducted by Health Centric Marketing Services, internal organizational forces have led to an increased focus on strategic marketing. Additionally, external environmental forces, such as managed care penetration and competitive pressures, have forced medical group practices to respond with an increased focus on marketing.[6]

Changes in the financing and delivery of health care continue to threaten the survival of medical group practices. The growth of managed care has intensified the struggle to maintain revenue and continues to threaten the viability of many medical groups. In order to survive, medical groups must be able to strategically plan and change direction quickly and constantly.

The ideas of strategic planning and marketing are not new; they have been utilized effectively in manufacturing and other service industries for decades. They have also been employed by larger health care systems, such as hospitals. The majority of medical group practices, however, have not committed the resources to strategically plan for the future. Instead, all but the largest of medical group practices continue to struggle to react and keep afloat in the turbulent and ever-changing waters of the health care market.

Strategic planning offers a path that shows medical practice executives how to achieve goals and objectives on a consistent basis.[7] Successful medical group practices will be those that embrace strategic planning and marketing, rather than those that accept incremental, reactive adjustments.

Knowledge Needs

WITHIN THE MEDICAL PRACTICE MANAGEMENT Body of Knowledge domain of Planning and Marketing are many essential skills and a knowledge base in which executives should demonstrate competency. Some of these skills have been discussed already, as they have been identified as the general competencies that all practice executives should possess: Professionalism, Leadership, Communication Skills, Organizational and Analytical Skills, and Technical/Professional Knowledge and Skills. In addition to these general competencies are those specific to planning and marketing: executives should be visionaries, risk-takers, aware of industry trends, customer-focused, tuned in to stakeholder needs, and one step ahead of the competition.

Practice executives must have a vision of the past, present, and – most important – future; and must succeed in communicating such a vision to others in a way that their followers adopt the vision as their own. Executives must not just see the vision themselves, they must have the ability to convince others to see it also. This is an important skill in planning and marketing. In planning, the vision of the practice (and executive) guides many of the goals and strategies; it sets the tone for where the practice would like to see itself in the future (e.g., providing the highest-quality care, being the leading specialty practice in the region, serving all who need care, and so forth). In marketing, this skill is equally important. If the practice executive has a vision for the practice, this can often be articulated into an effective marketing strategy.

Accepting that taking risks is an inherent part of the planning process is also a skill that is necessary for the practice executive's success in planning and marketing. Each decision – pursuing a strategy aimed at establishing a new practice site, offering a new service, hiring new partners – possesses a degree of risk. The practice executive should possess skills that allow for a degree of informed and appropriate risk-taking when it comes to planning and marketing.

The practice executive should have a broad knowledge of the current and future issues and trends taking place within the health care industry in general and in the community more specifically. This awareness will allow the executive to plan and market efficiently and effectively. It will also provide the executive with insight as to what the competition might be planning and what consumers will be requesting in the future.

Additional knowledge with regard to the needs of internal and external stakeholders will also help ensure success in planning and marketing. Internal stakeholders (e.g., physicians in the practice and clinical and business staff) and external stakeholders (e.g., customers/patients, the community in general, and other group practices) are vital to the success of each plan. Being aware of their needs and factoring these into the plans will yield support in implementing each plan.

Each of these skills can be seen as essential for the medical practice executive in the domain of Planning and Marketing. A deficiency in one or more should raise concern because serious pitfalls in planning and marketing may occur.

Overview of Planning and Marketing Tasks

■ TASK 1: **Develop strategic plans**

The health care environment is one of continuous change: change in reimbursement; change in financial and organizational oversight; change in leadership; change in policies, regulations, and standards; change in the health care needs and wants of the populations served. These changes can be further classified into the types of decisions the medical practice executive should make to "strategically" position the organization for success. Robert Shirley identified these decision areas as:

1. *Mission, vision, goals, and objectives* – The organization's purpose and aim for the future and the results it seeks to accomplish;

2. *Service area and stakeholder relationships* – The geographic service area and target market to be served and the relationships with internal and external bodies of influence;

3. *Program, service, and product mix* – The specific programs, services, and/or products to be offered to meet the needs of the service areas and stakeholders; and

4. *Competitive advantage* – The means by which the organization seeks to differentiate itself from other similar organizations.[8]

As illustrated in the case study earlier in this volume, these four decision areas are critical to achieving practice "differentiation." Medical practice executives should be able to address these changes and formulate plans in each of these decision areas in a manner that will position the practice to remain viable and successful. Overlooking or not anticipating such changes or decisions can be disastrous. Strategic planning is a tool that enables the executive to anticipate, prepare, and manage change and guide decision making strategically.

■ TASK 2: **Create business plans**

The medical group practice's strategic plan can serve as a useful foundation on which to base a more detailed and comprehensive business plan. A business plan precisely defines the practice, identifies its goals, and serves as its operational resume. It offers a practice a means to accomplish the goals it establishes in its strategic plan, such as securing capital, marketing the practice's services, recruiting new employees, or planning for growth.[9] The business plan also assists the medical practice executive in allocating resources and making good business decisions. Like the strategic plan, the business plan should be specific, informative, and future-oriented.

Essentially, the practice's business plan needs to address:

1. The practice's current position with regard to clientele, services being offered, competition, and trends within the specialty and field;

2. Where the practice envisions itself in one to three years in terms of specific goals; and

3. What it will take to move the practice from its current position to its desired position – in particular, to deal with the trends and the competitors.

In particular, the executive of any medical group practice that is beginning or extending a venture (e.g., adding a service, recruiting new partners, opening an additional location, or merging with or acquiring another practice) that will consume significant resources (money, energy, and/or time) and that is expected to return a profit, should take the time to complete a business plan.

■ TASK 3: **Create marketing plans**

In addition to the strategic plan and business plan, many organizations find it useful to also develop a marketing plan. The marketing plan incorporates much of the research of the two previous plans, but shifts the focus to the external environment. The medical practice executive should identify segments, select the target market, and position and develop the 4Ps (product, price, promotion, place) expected from marketers.

At the strategic marketing plan level, the medical practice executive should be scanning the environment, pondering what is happening, and looking for emerging or robust market segments to be considered as target markets. The outcomes of such plans are clearly identified target markets and the strategies that will meet their needs, as identified in the marketing analysis. Marketing plan objectives are typically on the level of sales, profit, return on investment (ROI), or, for the larger practice, market share.

■ TASK 4: **Monitor and evaluate effectiveness of strategic, business, and marketing plan activities**

It is not enough to simply develop strategic, business, and marketing plans. But all too often, this is what occurs. Many a practice will go through the planning processes only to create documents that collect dust on the shelf after they are completed. Monitoring and evaluating the planning activities and status of implementation of each plan is – for many practices – as important as identifying the goals and strategies compiled in each plan. These activities enhance the effectiveness of the plans by establishing clear links between past, present, and future strategies and results. With a systematic method to compare actual performance to planned performance, the medical practice executive can determine the effectiveness of the actions.

The planning process remains incomplete until the results or impacts of the efforts are evaluated. Unfortunately, the importance of this particular procedure is often underestimated. By evaluating the results of past goals or activities, the medical practice executive will be in a more favorable position to gain and share invaluable experiences. In addition, the executive will improve not only the planning process, but ultimately his or her own personal skills as an evaluator and program planner.

Monitoring and evaluation can help the practice manager to extract, from past and ongoing activities, relevant information that can subsequently be used as the basis for fine-tuning strategies, reorienting strategic directions, and planning. Without monitoring and evaluation, it would be impossible to assess if strategies were going in the right direction, whether progress and success could be declared, and how future efforts might be improved. A formal process for monitoring and evaluating performance also increases the accountability of the medical practice and practice executive in implementing the outcomes and strategies of the various plans.

■ TASK 5: **Pursue and establish partnerships and strategic alliances**

Alliances are not new to health care; rather, they have been a part of the medical group practice scene for years. To survive today's tumultuous health care market, it is vital that organizations strategically position themselves by forming alliances. Alliances are a form of cooperative arrangement between two or more physician groups or between physicians and hospitals.[10] Strategic alliances are the basis of a popular strategy that allows two or more organizations to pool resources to gain access to up-to-date technology and maintain competitive advantage in hypercompetitive environments, such as health care.[11]

The medical practice executive is ultimately responsible for negotiating contracts, forming alliances, and establishing partnerships. These responsibilities require and presume discretionary authority and, as a condition of this authority, the practice executive owes the organization the duty of loyalty.[12] As such, the executive must be cognizant of the needs of not only the shareowners, but all of the stakeholders of the firm. Consequently, the practice executive has a moral and legal obligation to deal openly and honestly with the firm's various stakeholders.

The success of a medical group practice rests with the practice executive's ability to forge alliances in which diverse individuals and interests collaborate to leverage resources for the benefit of two or more organizations. This task has been developed in response to these concerns and needs. The guidelines for this task are intended to make the practice executive aware of the management processes surrounding alliances and partnerships.

■ TASK 6: Develop and implement community outreach, public relations, and customer relations programs

To prosper in today's health care market, organizations need to build trust and commitment within the community and among the customers they serve. To do so, medical practice executives need to engage in open and frequent communication with members of the community in which they operate.[13] To be effective, the medical practice executive must employ a long-term strategy that is driven by commitment, continuity, and consistency so that the relationship with the community can be sustained.[14]

Commitment requires that individual organizations select and provide services and programs that are beneficial to the community and also commit practice resources to ensure that these efforts can be maintained. To ensure continuity, it is critical that medical practice executives actively manage the relationship with the community and patients on an ongoing basis to ensure long-term survival.

Another important facet of developing community and customer programs is consistency. The best way to ensure consistency is through written policy so that new employees can be trained and oriented appropriately. Otherwise, staff and administrator turnover will cripple any and all attempts to build consistency and continuity.

Developing programs aimed at the community and the customer is an essential part of any medical practice executive's marketing strategy. This task involves several strategies that can be employed by medical group practices; however, not all strategies are applicable to every situation.

TASK 1 **Develop Strategic Plans**

■ Strategic Planning Defined

▶ Planning is a formalized procedure to produce an articulated result, in the form of an integrated system of decisions. Thinking about and attempting to control the future are important components of planning.[15]

▶ Planning is required when the future state we desire involves a set of interdependent decisions; that is a system of decisions.[16]

▶ [Strategy] determines and reveals the organizational purpose in terms of long-term objectives, action programs, and resource allocation priorities; attempts to achieve a long-term sustainable advantage in each of its businesses by responding appropriately to the opportunities and threats in the firm's environment, and the strengths and weaknesses of the organization; identifies the distinct managerial tasks at the corporate, business, and functional levels; is a coherent, unifying, and integrative pattern of decisions; defines the nature of the economic and non-economic contributions it intends to make to its stakeholders; is an expression of the strategic intent of the organization; is aimed at developing and nurturing the core competencies of the firm; and is a means for investing selectively in tangible and intangible resources to develop the capabilities that assure a sustainable competitive advantage.[17]

▶ Strategic planning is a complex and ongoing process of organizational change. It is a disciplined effort to produce fundamental decisions and actions that shape and guide what an organization is, what it does, and why it does it, with a focus on the future.[18]

■ Differences between Conventional Planning and Strategic Planning

One of the major differences between conventional planning and strategic planning is that "conventional planning tends to be oriented toward looking at problems based on current understanding, or an inside-out mind-set. Strategic planning requires an understanding of the nature of the issue, and then finding of an appropriate response, or an outside-in mind-set."[19]

Long-range planning is a projection from the present or an extrapolation from the past. It also tends to be numbers-driven. Strategic planning, on the other hand, builds on anticipated future trends, data, and competitive assumptions and tends to be idea-driven; it seeks to provide a clear organizational vision or focus. If, for example, a medical practice finds through its planning research that its community is fast becoming a Mecca for retiring seniors, the group would be wise to strategically add certain types of staff or services over the coming years that would be attractive to this population.

■ The Strategic Planning Process: Who, What, When, Where, Why, and How?

Before initiating the planning process, the organization must plan to plan. Key concepts – such as *who* should be involved in the planning process, *what* the goal or direction of the planning process is, *when* and *where* planning should take place, *why* the organization is planning, and *how* it will all be accomplished – need to be addressed prior to beginning the planning process.

Who?

One of the most detrimental mistakes a medical group practice can make is putting the planning process solely in the hands of the administrator, with little involvement from others within, or even outside of, the organization. The administrator and board chair should be included in the planning group, and should drive the development and implementation of the plan, but their buy-in and participation, although essential for the plan to come to fruition, should take on the role of facilitator vs. active participant. The same can be said for the role of the entire board. Demonstrated support through encouragement and motivation, meeting attendance, and resource allocation (time, space, financial) are the main roles of the administrator and board members.

The coordination and facilitation of strategic planning in general should be designated as the responsibility of a key manager, and development of the strategy should be a line job, with each manager responsible for the strategic implications of his or her decisions.[20] The rationale for this is that the managers and staff are more "in touch" with the activities that take place within their areas because they are firsthand responders. Who better to identify areas of change than those who have identified the need for it?

However, in some cases, consideration should be given to hiring a facilitator or consultant from outside of the organization to lead the strategic planning process before resting the leadership responsibility on one of the managers or staff. If any of the following is a concern, outside assistance may be warranted:

1. If this is the organization's initial attempt at conducting strategic planning;

2. If planning efforts have been unsuccessful in the past;

3. If there appears to be a wide range of ideas and/or concerns among organization members about strategic planning and current organizational issues to be addressed in the plan;

4. If the members believe there is no one in the organization who has sufficient facilitation skills;

5. If no one in the organization is committed to facilitating strategic planning for the organization;

6. If leaders believe that an inside facilitator will either inhibit participation from others or will not have the opportunity to fully participate in planning themselves, and/or

7. If leaders want an objective voice (e.g., someone who is not likely to have strong predispositions about the organization's strategic direction issues and ideas).[21]

Once it has been determined who will be facilitating the strategic planning process, the planning team should be formed. The first step in establishing the team is to identify its membership. For example, who will be directly involved in planning, who will provide key information to the process, who will review the plan, who will authorize the plan, and who will lead implementation of the plan. There should be at least one person appointed to the team who ultimately has authority to make strategic decisions (e.g., to select which goals will be achieved and how). The composition of the team should also ensure that as many stakeholders as possible, internal and external, are involved in the planning process. Internal stakeholders, such as physicians, clinical staff, and clerical staff, should be well represented. Each will bring a different perspective to the process. It is also likely that external stakeholders, such as patients, vendors/suppliers, and contract staff, may have valuable input at some point in the planning process, so it is a good idea to include them when that point arises. A word of caution, however – many of these "external" stakeholders may also share this type of relationship with the organization's competitors. Sometimes, it may be wise to communicate the confidentiality of meetings and possibly ask participants to sign nondisclosure agreements.

There is no "ideal" number of members for the strategic planning team. If the organization is very small, all employees may be involved; if the organization is large, a representative from each division, area, or department may be selected. Therefore, team membership could range from 2 to 50 representatives. Subcommittees should be used to manage team membership when it grows to larger than 20. This will ensure that all voices are heard throughout the process.

What and Why?

Once the planning team has been established, it is important to ensure that the team understands what its charter is, why the team has been tasked with it, and why the charter is important to and valued by the organization. There must be buy-in from all involved to ensure a successful planning process and the development and implementation of a plan that will assist the organization in managing change and in its decision making for the future. Instilling a sense of ownership in the organization and bringing together everyone's best and most reasoned efforts have important value in building a consensus about where an organization is going. It also provides a clearer focus of organization, producing more efficiency and effectiveness, and in turn increasing productivity.

When and Where?

The next step is to determine the number of meetings the committee should have. This will depend on whether the organization has done planning before, how many strategic issues and goals the organization faces, whether the culture of the organization prefers short or long meetings, and how much time the organization is willing to commit to strategic planning.[22]

Most organizations attempt to complete the strategic planning in two to three months, with meetings every few weeks. This is a good range – any longer and the momentum possibly will be lost and the planning effort may fall apart. An effective way to initiate the planning process is to host an off-site retreat for one or two days, as it provides a change of pace and encourages participants to think outside the box – or outside the office. Dedicating this much time up front reinforces the importance of the process and the support by administration. It also allows the equivalent of months of one-hour meetings to be conducted in one or two days, in an uninterrupted fashion.

How?

The final step in the planning-to-plan process is to provide the team with the tools and resources it needs to develop, implement, and maintain the plan. Adequate resources in the form of supplies (white board, markers, flip charts, paper, etc.), time, money, and creative freedom need to be dedicated to this task. If this is a new undertaking within the organization, dedicating funds to be used for hiring a facilitator or consultant, or sending staff to training, is recommended. The leader of this initiative needs to understand the steps involved and needs to be able to facilitate the completion of each step in the process.

Organizational Culture

An additional consideration at this stage is the culture of the organization. Although there is not one standard definition of organizational culture, "the way we do things around here" is an efficient and frequently cited commonsense definition of culture. Many of the problems confronting administrators can be traced to their inability to analyze and evaluate organizational cultures. When trying to implement new strategies or a strategic plan, medical practice executives will often discover that their strategies will fail if they are inconsistent with the organization's culture.

Schein presents five guidelines for the administrator when addressing organizational culture:

1. Don't oversimplify culture or confuse it with climate, values, or corporate philosophy. Culture *underlies* and largely *determines* these other variables. Trying to change values or climate without getting at the underlying culture will be a futile effort.

2. Don't label culture as solely a human resources (read "touchy-feely") aspect of an organization, affecting only its human side. The impact of culture goes far beyond the human side of the organization to affect and influence its basic mission and goals.

3. Don't assume that the leader can manipulate culture just as s/he can control many other aspects of the organization. Culture, because it is largely determined and controlled by the members of the organization, and not the leaders, is

different. Culture may end up controlling the leader rather than being controlled by the leader!

4. Don't assume that there is a "right or wrong" culture, or that a strong culture is better than a weak one. It should be apparent that different cultures may fit different organizations and their environments, and that the desirability of a strong culture depends on how well it supports the organization's strategic goals and objectives.

5. Don't assume that all the aspects of an organization's culture are important, or will have a major impact on the functioning of the organization. Some elements of an organization's culture may have little impact on its functioning, and the leader must distinguish which elements are important, and focus on those.[23]

An understanding of culture, and how to transform it, is a crucial skill for administrators trying to achieve strategic outcomes. Due to their position in the organization, administrators are best situated to see the dynamics of the culture, such as what should remain and what needs transformation. This is the essence of strategic success.

■ Components of the Strategic Plan

The strategic plan, as briefly discussed earlier, is "a disciplined effort to produce fundamental decisions and actions that shape and guide what an organization is, what it does, and why it does it, with a focus on the future."[24] To accomplish this goal, several activities must take place in a sequential order, related to mission, vision, values, goals, and objectives.

Mission

The first step in the strategic planning process is to define the medical group practice's mission – its purpose or reason for being. This is usually illustrated in a mission and/or vision statement for the practice, the values of the practice, and in the practice's goals and objectives. If the practice cannot clearly articulate what its purpose is, what it values, and in what direction it is headed in the future, then the remaining steps in the planning process cannot be addressed. In other words, *all* planning for the organization hinges on this first step.

The mission of an organization is the organization's precise statement of purpose. It helps keep management focused on preserving or strengthening the organization's unique competitive niche. The mission assists in transforming ideas into action. It can also prevent panic and unwise marketing or spending responses to meet an indirect thrust by competitors. Most organizations have limited resources, and a mission statement is a constant reminder of where those limited resources should be focused. Another advantage of a mission statement is that it promotes unity within the organization – it elicits an emotional, motivational response in company employees. This, in turn, creates a culture that is less resistant to change. Focusing on the most important purposes of an organization also brings clarity to expectations, again strengthening the culture of the organization. Developing a mission statement is a challenging process; however, the benefits realized make it worth the effort.

The best mission statements use simple speech with no technical jargon and no embellishment, and can be transferred into individual action every day. For example, the mission statement of MGMA is "to continually improve the performance of medical group practice professionals and the organizations they represent" – MGMA comes right out and says something. So does Merck: "We are in the business of preserving and improving human life"; and Disney: "To use our imagination to bring happiness to millions of people."[25]

The most successful missions are measurable, definable, and actionable project statements with emotional appeal that everyone knows and can act upon. A mission such as "to be the best health care provider in the world" sounds good for a medical group practice, but a simple mission statement, such as the one Pepsi used at one point – "beat Coke!" – is even better because it is a statement that can be measured every day by every employee. Mission statements can also affect company strategies and tactics. If Pepsi were to change its mission to "beat Czech Cola," different strategies would be called for, along with different geographic tactics in sales, advertising, and distribution.

Formulating a mission statement is best accomplished by asking the planning team a few key questions: What is our main function? Why do we exist? Whom do we serve? What do we value? How are we unique? As these questions are evaluated, a mission statement will start to evolve.

Vision

The vision statement of an organization outlines what an organization wants to be. It is future-oriented, inspirational, and ambitious; however, it is also realistic and achievable. Typically, a vision is "more important as a guide to implementing strategy than it is to formulating it."[26] This is because strategy development is driven by what the organization is trying to accomplish – the organization's purpose(s). A mission statement answers the questions: Why do we exist? What business are we in? What do we value? A vision, however, is more encompassing. It answers the question: What does the organization look like as it effectively carries out its mission? It is the pursuit of this image of success that really motivates people to work together.

Building on the previous mission statement examples, the visions of those organizations are as follows:

- MGMA's vision (MGMA-Missouri): "MGMA-MO aspires to be the recognized source of professional enrichment for health care managers in Missouri."

- PepsiCo's vision: "Our responsibility is to continually improve all aspects of the world in which we operate – environment, social, economic – creating a better tomorrow than today."

- Merck's vision: "Our shared vision is to discover, develop and deliver innovative pharmaceutical products that meet a true need and make a real difference to people's lives."
- Disney's vision: "We make people happy."

A vision should challenge and inspire the practice to achieve its mission, just as these examples have illustrated. A vision should orient the practice's energies and serve as a guide to action. It should also be consistent with the practice's values.

Values

Values represent the core priorities in the organization's culture, including what drives members' priorities and how they truly act in the organization. Values represent the organization's highest priorities and deeply held driving forces. They are statements about how the organization will value customers, suppliers, and the internal community. Value statements describe actions that are the living enactment of the fundamental values held by most individuals within the organization. Values are increasingly important in strategic planning. They often drive the intent and direction for the planning team.[27]

In developing a value statement, team members may use methods ranging from highly analytical and rational to highly creative and divergent, such as focused discussions, divergent experiences around daydreams, and sharing stories.[28] The Nominal Group Technique (NGT) is an effective tool to use in developing the organization's value statement. A few of the advantages to using this technique, rather than focus groups or roundtable discussions during scheduled meetings, are that NGT balances participation across members and produces a greater number of ideas, and more creative ideas, than traditional interacting groups. The NGT process, as it applies to developing a statement of values for the organization, is presented in a flowchart in Exhibit 1.

No matter what method is chosen for formulating the values statement for the organization, four to six core values from which the organization would like to operate should be selected. In select-

EXHIBIT 1.
Flowchart of Nominal Group Technique steps

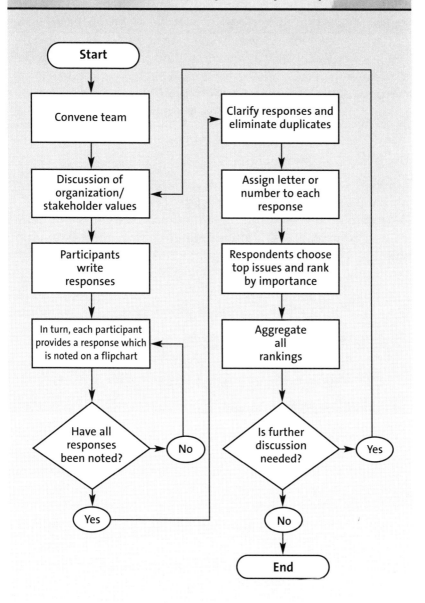

ing these values, internal (e.g., staff, physicians) and external (e.g., patients, payers, vendors, competitors, community) stakeholders' values should be considered. Attention should be given to any differences observed between the organization's preferred values and its true values (the values actually reflected by members' behaviors in the organization). For example, if patient service and satisfaction is a chosen value, is the front desk staff empowered to schedule appointments based on the patient's schedule or based solely on the physician's schedule? Are office hours convenient for working parents, including evening and weekend hours?

Goals and Objectives

The goals and objectives of the organization are the next items that need to be developed. However, before this can be accomplished, it is important to assess the organization's internal environment (strengths, weaknesses) and external environment (opportunities, threats). This type of assessment of the organization's strategic environment is referred to as a SWOT analysis, referring to the organization's strengths, weaknesses, opportunities, and threats. The two key questions a SWOT analysis addresses are:

1. What are the significant issues that the group practice faces today?

2. How should the group practice attend to these issues?

An example of a SWOT analysis is presented in Exhibit 2.

The SWOT analysis will reveal where the medical group practice should focus its resources, and the practice's goals and objectives (e.g., strategies) should arise from this. For example, if one of the practice's *weaknesses* is in providing geriatric care and a physician is retiring from the practice, a goal could be structured around the *opportunity* of recruiting a physician who specializes in geriatric care and expanding the practice to meet the needs of this growing population. The practice thus would be overcoming its weakness by pursuing an opportunity.

EXHIBIT 2.

Strategic plan SWOT analysis

INTERNAL FACTORS	EXTERNAL FORCES
Strengths	**Opportunities**
What does your practice do well? ■ In this cell, the internal strengths of the practice should be highlighted. Strengths can relate to the practice at large, to the environment, to perceptions, and to people. "People" elements include the skills, capabilities, and knowledge of participants.	*Where are the opportunities for your practice?* ■ In this cell, the external opportunities for the practice should be highlighted. Opportunities can entail socioeconomic, environmental, and demographic factors.
Weaknesses	**Threats**
What part of your practice needs improvement? ■ In this cell, the internal weaknesses of the practice are identified. This should include an honest appraisal of how things are in the practice. It is not uncommon for "people" problems to emerge as major weaknesses (e.g., poor communication, lack of leadership, little trust, etc.).	*What is happening in your area that could threaten your practice?* ■ In this cell, the external threats for the practice are identified. Threats are events that may, with a change of emphasis or perception, have an adverse impact on the practice. The same factors may emerge as both a threat and an opportunity.

Goals and objectives for the practice need to be SMART – specific, measurable, attainable, realistic, and tangible. Specific goals and objectives are more likely to be accomplished than general ones. A general goal would be to "recruit a new physician." Using our previous example, a specific goal would be to "recruit a physician who specializes in geriatric medicine." Without a means of measuring the goals and objectives (e.g., setting a deadline date, a percentage to improve, a number to achieve), knowing when they are accomplished can become difficult. For example, a goal that states, "We will recruit two new physicians – one geriatric specialist and one generalist – by March 2007," is more likely to be understood and accomplished than a goal that simply states "We will recruit new physicians for the practice." When goals and objectives are attainable and realistic, they are set at a level that practices can and will work toward achieving. Goals and objectives are tangible when they can be experienced with one of the senses – taste, touch, smell, sight, or hearing. When goals and objectives are tangible, making them specific and measurable, there is a better chance of attaining them.

■ Summary

The strategic planning process is a dynamic one that involves most internal stakeholders within a practice as well as many external stakeholders. Involvement takes:

- The form of strategic planning team membership;
- Internal and external data collection and analysis;
- Development of the practice's mission, vision, values, goals, and objectives; and
- Writing, implementing, and maintaining the strategic plan.

Each component is vital for the practice to strategically position itself for the future, and the medical practice executive should make sure that adequate support (e.g., administrator, physicians, board, and staff buy-in) and resources (e.g., time, money, and staff) are allocated to ensure this.

TASK 2 **Create Business Plans**

TO BE EFFECTIVE in today's market, medical group practices should adopt some of the same tools used in other successful "businesses," including strategic plans, marketing plans, and business plans. Whereas, as Task 1 shows, the strategic plan tends to focus on trends and competition, a business plan addresses the practice's resources, such as the breadth and depth of the practice, technological expertise, and service delivery capabilities, among other assets. The marketing plan, addressed in Task 3, focuses on customers – patients, other physicians and groups, payers, vendors, and the community at large.

■ Selecting a Type of Plan

There are four basic types of business plans, each with a unique purpose and audience:

1. Start-up business plan;
2. Ongoing financial business plan;
3. Operational business plan; and
4. Bank-financing plan.

Start-up Business Plan

Practices that are seeking funds to help start a new venture, such as opening a second office or purchasing equipment to offer new services, need to complete a start-up business plan. This type of plan is used to convince potential investors to provide the practice with the necessary capital to pursue this new venture. A start-up plan is sometimes referred to as an "idea" plan. In this type of plan, the practice would brainstorm and then outline the venture: What problem, weakness, or opportunity is the practice addressing through this plan? How does this new venture solve the problem? Why is this solution better than others? How will it be marketed? What resources are required to make it happen? The purpose of this type of plan is to allow the practice to see whether the venture is worth undertaking. If so, the practice can use the plan to recruit stakeholders who share its vision and bring them onboard for the new venture.

Ongoing Financial Business Plan

Established practices that are seeking financial support may complete an ongoing financial business plan. This type of plan will also allow potential lending sources to view the practice's ongoing financial status, risk, past and future spending habits, and prospects before committing funds. Because the practice is established, financials from more than one year can be trended.

Operational Business Plan

A third type of plan is the operational business plan, the most detailed of the plans. It documents exact operation plans for the practice through items such as the detailed operating budget, detailed market and competitor research and analysis, product design specs, sales prospect lists, partner acquisition strategies, intellectual property strategies, and anything else that guides the group's growth.

Bank-Financing Plan

The final type of business plan is the bank-financing plan, used when a practice is trying to obtain a bank loan. Perhaps the group would like to offer a new ancillary service that requires significant capital (e.g., lab services, radiology, etc.). Bank funding is usually available only if the practice either has a solid operating history with positive cash flows or can put up collateral to cover the loan (for a start-up, this means something of great value, such as a house). The bank-financing plan focuses on persuading the banker that the practice can satisfy these needs through historical financial ratios, assets, and so forth.

■ Getting Started

Before writing a business plan, the medical practice executive should consider four core questions:

1. **What** service or product does the practice provide and what needs does it fill?

2. **Who** are the potential customers for the practice's service(s) and why will they choose the practice for them?

3. **How** will the practice reach its potential customers?

4. **Where** will the practice get the financial resources to start new endeavors, such as new products or services?

The preparation of a written business plan is not the end result of the planning process. The realization of that plan is the ultimate goal. However, the writing of the plan is an important intermediate stage – *fail to plan can mean plan to fail.* For an established practice, it demonstrates that careful consideration has been given to the practice's development; and for a start-up, it shows that the entrepreneur has done his or her homework.

A formal business plan is just as important for an established practice, irrespective of its size, as it is for a start-up practice. It serves four critical functions:

1. Helps a practice to clarify, focus, and research its planned future development and prospects.

2. Provides a considered and logical framework within which a

practice can develop and pursue business strategies over the next three to five years.

3. Serves as a basis for discussion with third parties such as shareholders, agencies, banks, and investors.

4. Offers a benchmark against which actual practice performance can be measured and reviewed.

■ Business Plan Components

Five main components are typically found in every business plan: (1) an executive summary, (2) a business section, (3) a market analysis section, (4) a financial section, and (5) a management section.

Executive Summary

Every business plan begins with an executive summary. The executive summary is the "first impression" of the practice that you give to the reader, be it a potential lender, partner, or investor. The cliché "You never have a second chance to make a good first impression" applies here because the success of the plan can often depend on the executive summary. The executive summary briefly, yet accurately, responds to the five core questions – the who, what, when, where, and how of the venture. It also provides a succinct overview of each of the other main components of the plan (e.g., business, market analysis, financials, and management) as well as components from the strategic plan (mission, vision, values, and goals and objectives). The executive summary answers the questions: Where is the practice going? What will it look like when it gets there? What is the present situation in the community (and for larger groups – across the country) and how does it affect the practice? What is the status of the practice's products or services? What about its finances? What management is in place? Who needs to be hired or recruited? The executive summary should be written *after* the business plan has been completed.

Business Section

The second component of the business plan is the business section. This section discusses the practice's structure, management, staffing, operations, and business relationships. This section usually begins with a brief description of the industry as it looks today, as well as how it will look in the future. Information on all the various markets within the industry, including any new products or developments that will benefit or adversely affect the practice, also should be discussed. An explanation of the structure – general or limited partnership, sole proprietorship, or corporation, for example – should be stated, as well as the practice's legal form, who its principals are, and what they will bring to the venture.

After the description of the practice's business comes an explanation of the products or services the practice intends to market. The product/services description statement should be complete enough to give a clear idea of the practice's intentions. Emphasis should be given to any unique features or variations from concepts that can typically be found in the industry. Examples of where a practice's unique features can be promoted might include sponsoring a booth at a county fair providing free blood pressure and cholesterol screening, or physicians attending disease-specific support groups (congenital heart, diabetes, etc.) and providing information and, often more importantly, answering patient and family member's questions.

Market Analysis Section

The next section of the business plan provides a market analysis, which is essentially a summary of the practice's marketing plan. The market analysis demonstrates the demand for the practice's products or services, the proposed market, and trends within the industry. In addition, it describes the practice's pricing plan and policies. This section helps the practice understand and define its market, the demographics and psychographics of its target customers, competitor's products or services, and both business and environmental risks.

For marketing to be effective, the medical group practice should have a differentiable market position that can be held out to the potential client in a verifiable, demonstrable way. Marketing activities in a business plan must be based on a foundation of practice management activities to truly differentiate the practice.[29] Practice management activities in a business plan include steps such as increasing the practice's patient base or capabilities through recruiting additional physicians, developing new products or services, developing in-depth industry knowledge (by which the practice will be known as being expert within a particular specialty), and so forth.[30]

The world might "beat a path to your door," but only if people know who you are, what you've got, and where to find you. Thus, the market analysis also includes the practice's advertising and promotion, pricing and profitability, selling tactics, distribution, public relations, and business relationships.[31] A key component of the market analysis section that affects everything the practice does throughout its business is summarized in the question: How will the practice use an investor's money to efficiently market to its customers?

Financial Section

The next section of the business plan comprises the financials of the practice. This section demonstrates that the practice is as committed to its business venture as it expects those reading the business plan to be. The practice's capital requirements and profit potential are analyzed and demonstrated here. This is accomplished through numerous financial statements, often based on a modified accrual accounting system that also takes into consideration "non-cash" items (e.g., capital expenditures, such as equipment or building leases). This is done in an effort to best reflect the financial health of the practice.

Accounting Methods

Accrual-based accounting systems record financial situations based on events that change the net worth of the practice (the amount owed to the practice less the amount the practice owes others). Standard practice is to record and recognize revenues when they become available and measurable (i.e., known). The term "available" means collectible within the current period or soon enough thereafter to be used to pay the liabilities of the current period. Expenditures, if measurable, are recorded in the accounting period in which the liabilities are incurred. An exception is unmatured interest on general long-term debt, which should be recorded when it is due.

This differs from cash-based accounting, used less often in medical practice management. In cash-based accounting, income and expenses are recognized only when cash is received or paid out. Cash-based accounting also defers all credit transactions to a later date. It is more conservative for the practice in that it does not record revenue until cash receipt. In a growing practice this results in a lower income bottom line compared to accrual-based accounting.

Financial statements should be prepared on the modified accrual-basis to show the amount and source of personal funds the practice is contributing, the amount of capital needed, and the practice's plan to repay this debt. All pertinent financial worksheets should be included in this section: income statement, a break-even worksheet, projected cash flow statements, and a balance sheet. A review of the practice's return on investment and discounted cash-flow value should also be completed.

Income Statement

The income statement is a report on the proposed or current business's cash-generating ability. The income statement illustrates just how much the practice makes or loses during the year by subtracting cost of goods and expenses from revenue to arrive at a net result – which is either a profit or a loss. For a business plan, the income statement should be generated on a monthly basis during the first year, quarterly for the second, and annually for each year thereafter. Following the income statement is a note analyzing the statement. The analysis statement should be very short, emphasizing key points within the income statement.[32]

Break-Even Worksheet

The break-even worksheet computes the break-even point and sales level needed to earn a given profit by analyzing relationships between fixed costs, variable costs per unit, quantity, price, and profit. This calculation is completed by first filling in all of the practice's expected fixed monthly expenses; these are expenses that will not change, regardless of the amount of services provided (how much is "sold"). These will add up to the practice's total fixed costs. The next step is to divide the total monthly fixed costs by the gross profit per unit. The result of this calculation is the break-even point.

The practice will operate at a loss until it reaches the break-even point (that is, total costs = total revenues).

Cash Flow Statement

The cash flow statement shows how much cash will be needed to meet obligations, when it is going to be required, and what the source will be. It shows a schedule of the money coming into the practice and expenses that need to be paid out. The result is the profit or loss at the end of the month or year. If the practice runs a loss on its cash flow statement, it is a strong indicator that the practice will need additional cash to meet expenses.[33]

The cash flow statement also should be prepared on a monthly basis during the first year, on a quarterly basis during the second year, and on an annual basis thereafter. As with the income statement, the cash flow statement should be presented in a short summary in the business plan covering the key points derived from the cash flow statement.[34]

Balance Sheet

The last financial statement needed for the business plan is the balance sheet. Like the income and cash flow statements, the balance sheet uses information from all of the financial models developed in earlier sections of the business plan; however, unlike the previous statements, the balance sheet is generated solely on an annual basis for the business plan and is, more or less, a summary of all the preceding financial information broken down into three areas: (1) assets; (2) liabilities; and (3) equity.[35]

Assets are classified as current, long-term, or fixed assets. Current assets are those that will be converted to cash or will be used by the practice in a year or less, including cash, accounts receivable, inventory, and supplies. Long-term assets are those that will last more than one year, such as capital equipment, property, and investments. Fixed assets are similar to long-term assets, and include property, building structures, and so forth.

Like assets, liabilities are classified as current or long-term. If the debts are due in one year or less, they are classified as current liabilities; if they are due in more than one year, they are long-term liabilities. Examples of current liabilities are accounts payable, accrued liabilities, and taxes; long-term liabilities include payables in the forms of bonds, notes, and mortgages.

The final portion of the balance sheet is the practice's equity, which is the difference between its total assets and total liabilities. The amount of equity the practice has is used by investors when evaluating the company to determine the amount of capital they think they can safely invest in the business.

In the business plan, an analysis statement for the balance sheet should be created just as was done for the income and cash flow statements. The analysis of the balance sheet should be kept short and cover key points about the practice.

Return on Investment and Discounted Cash Flow

Two types of valuation methods typically found in business plans include return on investment and discounted cash flow. ROI is a measure of the practice's ability to use its assets to generate additional value for shareholders. It is used to determine whether a proposed investment is reasonable and how well this investment will repay the shareholder. It is calculated as the ratio of the amount gained (net profit or net loss) divided by net worth and expressed as a percentage. If a group practice has immediate objectives such as getting market revenue share, building infrastructure, or positioning itself for sale, an ROI might be measured in terms of meeting one or more of these objectives rather than in immediate profit or cost saving.

Discounted cash flow expresses how much a practice is worth today based on what it will earn in the future. It informs shareholders of their expected rate of return, given the amount invested and the practice's financial projections, and how much equity they will receive for the investment. It is a fairly accurate measure because it discounts, or adjusts, cash flows (projected ups and downs of revenue over a period of time) by a rate that is acceptable to the shareholder to account for risk and the time the investor must wait for a return.

Each of these methods is valuable to the business plan. The underlying idea of these valuation methods is that money today is worth more than money a year, or five years, or ten years, etc., from now because money in hand can be invested to earn interest and there is no risk you may not receive it in the future; it follows the adage "time value of money."

Risk Tolerance

The risk tolerance of the practice – its attitude toward accepting risk – plays a significant role in its financial planning. Risk tolerance is not something that can be measured, but asking a few questions can help the practice determine whether it is conservative, moderate, or aggressive in its financial makeup. A practice that is unfamiliar with investing, fearful of asset loss, or prefers saving to investing could be classified as having a rather conservative tolerance for risk. Conversely, a practice that is comfortable with long-term goal investing, that can withstand short-term losses, and that is also comfortable with the turbulent nature of investing is aggressively risk-tolerant. A practice that is somewhat in the middle of these extremes is classified as moderately risk tolerant.

Shareholders also vary in their levels of risk tolerance and want to be compensated for their risk; sound financial management and planning, along with the use of valuation strategies, allow this to occur.

Management Section

A discussion of the practice's management is the final piece of its business plan. This includes a description of the practice's organizational structure and administrative team (including resumes and biographies) as well as staffing projection data for the near future.

The goal of this section is to demonstrate how the practice and its administration are uniquely qualified and capable of achieving success. In particular, the following questions should be answered: Can the practice relate to the community and draw customers for its services from it? Can the practice deliver what these customers really want? Is the practice's administrative team qualified to do this?

The management section of the business plan is really a mini-interview with the practice's administration to assure an investor, lender, or potential partner that it has lined up the right people to make the venture a success. This section is one of the most crucial of the entire business plan. The only thing that will ensure success is the day-to-day activity of qualified people who are in the "driver's seat" following a mapped plan toward a vision.[36]

■ Summary

A business plan should be a realistic view of the expectations and long-term objectives for an established practice or a new venture to be undertaken by the practice. It provides the framework within which the practice must operate and, ultimately, succeed or fail. For a medical practice seeking external support, the plan is the most important sales document it is ever likely to produce because it could be the key to raising finances. Preparation of a comprehensive plan will not guarantee success in raising funds or mobilizing support, but lack of a sound plan will, almost certainly, ensure failure.[37]

TASK 3 **Create Marketing Plans**

> If the circus is coming to town and you
> paint a sign saying, "Circus is coming to Fair-
> grounds Sunday," that's Advertising. If you
> put the sign on the back of an elephant and
> walk him through town, that's a Promotion.
> If the elephant walks through the Mayor's
> flower bed, that's Publicity. If you can get
> the Mayor to laugh about it, that's Public
> Relations. And, if you planned the whole
> thing, that's Marketing!
>
> – *Author Unknown*

IN GENERAL, marketing activities are all those activities associated with identifying the particular wants and needs of a target market of customers, and then going about satisfying those customers better than the competition does. This involves doing market research on customers, analyzing their needs, and then making strategic decisions about product design, pricing, promotion, and distribution. This view is consistent with the following definition of marketing found in a popular marketing textbook: "Marketing is the process of planning and executing the conception, pricing, promotion, and distribution of ideas, goods, services, organizations, and events to create and maintain relationships that will satisfy individual and organizational objectives."[38]

■ Components of a Marketing Plan

To accomplish the "marketing" tasks identified in these definitions, a marketing plan similar to the strategic and business plans needs to be developed. This marketing plan follows a framework similar to those of the other plans: executive summary, situational analysis, marketing objectives, marketing strategies, and so on.

Executive Summary

The executive summary of the practice's marketing plan should address the following key elements:

- What are the dominant issues discovered in the practice's situational analysis?
- What are the key objectives the practice seeks to achieve – in the shortest possible form?
- What, in one or two sentences, is the practice's marketing strategy to achieve those objectives?
- What other concepts unique to the practice should be addressed?

Answers to these questions comprise the body of the marketing plan; therefore, the executive summary cannot be written until the plan has been completed. It will then serve as the "snapshot" of what the practice aims to accomplish with regard to strategic marketing.

Situational Analysis

The situational analysis investigates the macro- and microenvironment in a manner similar to the strategic plan. In fact, the same tool – the SWOT analysis – can be used in this stage of the marketing plan process. The practice should review its strategic plan's SWOT and then consider each of the SWOT's components from a consumer and market viewpoint: its external threats and opportunities, its internal strengths and weaknesses, including key success factors in the health care industry, and the practice's sustainable competitive advantage. Along with the strategic plan's SWOT analysis, a two-by-two matrix can be created to identify specific focus areas for the marketing plan: the macroenvironment, the internal practice environment, market analyses, and consumer analyses (see Exhibit 3).

Macroenvironmental analysis refers to continuous structured data collection and processing on a broad range of environmental factors, such as the economy, the governmental and legal environments, technology, and social culture. This allows the practice to act quickly, take advantage of opportunities before competitors do, and respond to environmental threats before significant damage is done. Scanning these macroenvironmental variables for threats and opportunities requires that each issue be rated on two dimensions:

EXHIBIT 3.

Marketing plan situational analysis two-by-two matrix

Macroenvironment	Market Analysis
What does your practice do well?	*Where are the opportunities for your practice?*
▪ Innovative leadership ▪ Good reputation	▪ Untapped market for new procedure ▪ Hiring new physician in practice ▪ Need for geriatric care in community
Consumer Analysis	**Internal Practice Analysis**
What part of your practice needs improvement?	*What is happening in your area that could threaten your practice?*
▪ High nurse turnover ▪ Location of practice ▪ Retiring physician ▪ Providing geriatric care	▪ New regulation ▪ Growing elderly population

(1) its potential impact on the practice, and (2) its likelihood of occurrence. Weighing its potential impact by its likelihood of occurrence provides an indication of its importance to the practice.

The mircoenvironmental, or internal, analysis seeks to uncover the resources of the practice that apply or can be applied to marketing efforts. These resources include money, time, people, and skills. What internal resources does the practice have that are underexploited? Finding these resources internally as opposed to having to seek them externally will provide countless benefits to the practice. Along with identification of resources, the practice's vision, mission, and goals (in particular, long-term goals/objectives, marketing goals/objectives, and financial goals/objectives) should be reviewed, and the culture of the practice should be considered. Each of these areas will have an impact on the marketing strategy of the practice.

A consumer analysis explores the demographic makeup of the practice's consumer base, but also delves a bit deeper into the consumers' purchasing and decision-making behaviors, their motivations and expectations, and loyalty segments. Who are the practice's current consumers? What brought them to the practice in the first place?

The final piece of the situational analysis is the market analysis. In the market analysis, the medical practice defines its market; identifies its market size and industry market trends; evaluates the market segmentation and strategic groups; and studies the competition's strengths, weaknesses, and market share. A tool often used in completing these tasks is Michael Porter's Five Forces Analysis,[39] which allows a systematic and structured analysis of market structure and competitive situation. The five forces consist of those forces close to a company that affect its ability to serve its customers and make a profit.

Four of the forces – the bargaining power of consumers, the bargaining power of suppliers, the threat of new entrants, and the threat of substitute products – combine with other variables to influence a fifth force, the level of competition in an industry. A change in any of the forces normally requires a practice to reassess the marketplace. Exhibit 4 illustrates Porter's Five Forces Analysis.

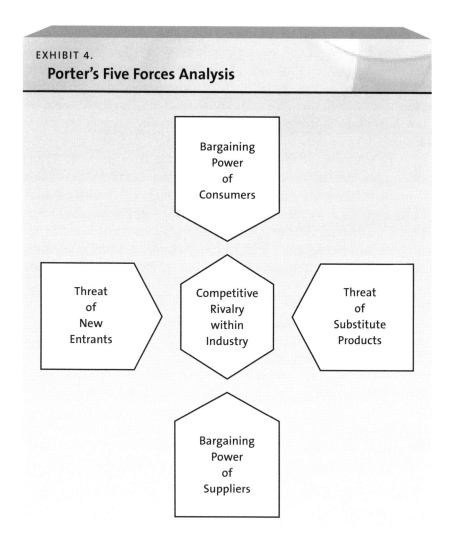

EXHIBIT 4.
Porter's Five Forces Analysis

The bargaining power of customers determines how much pressure on margins and volumes customers can impose. For example, customers will have high bargaining power when the ability to switch to an alternative product (e.g., a new prescription plan) is relatively simple and is not related to high costs, or when the customers have low margins and are price-sensitive (e.g., a small practice with few employees on a plan, but still needing a good price). The bargaining power of suppliers is similar. The term "suppliers" comprises all sources for inputs that are needed in order to provide goods or services. In such situations, the buying industry often faces a high pressure on margins from its suppliers. The relationship to powerful suppliers can potentially reduce strategic options for the practice.

When there is a threat of new entrants in the community that will compete with the practice, changes may occur in the major determinants of the market environment (e.g., market shares, prices, patient and staff loyalty) at any time. Remember that there is always a latent pressure for reaction and adjustment for existing competitors in the health care industry. A threat from substitutes exists if there are alternative products or services, or complementary products or services, with lower prices and/or higher quality that can be used for the same purpose. These competitors could potentially attract a significant proportion of market volume and consequently reduce the potential sales volume for existing practices. Competitive rivalry within the industry derives the intensity of competition among existing practices in the industry. High competitive pressure results in pressure on prices, margins, and profitability for every single company in the industry.

After the analysis of the current and potential future state of the five forces, the practice can search for options to influence these forces in its favor, thereby reducing the competitive forces' power.

Marketing Research

Marketing research is the next major task undertaken in the marketing plan process. The American Marketing Association defines marketing research as:

> ...the function that links the consumer, customer, and public to the marketer through information – information used to identify and define marketing opportunities and problems; generate, refine, and evaluate marketing actions; monitor marketing performance; and improve understanding of marketing as a process.

Market research specifies the information required to address these issues, designs the method for collecting information, manages and implements the data collection process, analyzes the results, and communicates the findings and their implications.[40]

The aim of marketing research is to find out the who, what, when, and where with regard to the practice's customers and services: Who are the customers? What services do they want? When do they want these services provided? Where do they want these services provided? Answers to these questions can reveal problems with current services as well as potential trends for the future. In addition to identifying the practice's customers and their preferences, market research should assist the practice in determining its market share and the effectiveness of its advertising and promotions.

Three general sources of market data can be gathered: (1) data already available externally (e.g., from the chamber of commerce, business coalitions, state trade organizations, and the U.S. Census Bureau); (2) data readily available internally (e.g., from employees, current customers, and company records and files); and (3) data that can be collected by and/or for the practice (e.g., through surveys, interviews, evaluation/response cards, customer feedback, and observations of competition). The practice executive should determine what form of market research will work best based on the value the practice will receive vs. the time and other resources it will need to invest to gain access to that information.

Market Strategy

With the market analysis completed, the next step in the marketing plan is to develop a market strategy, which details the broad plan to achieve the practice's objectives with regard to marketing. This may include using the information and data collected to determine which consumers' wants and needs are not being met by the practice or by the competition, or determining areas where new services or different services would capture new markets.[41]

In developing the marketing strategy, the practice needs to identify which segment it is "targeting." The target market is a specific group of consumers who have a want or need for the practice's services or products. For example, a dermatology practice is looking to market its new laser therapy to women, and has determined the target age range as 24 to 50 years of age. Target marketing allows the practice to reach, create awareness in, and influence the group of consumers (e.g., in this case, women aged 24 to 50) most likely to select its services while conserving resources and generating greater returns.

Market segmentation – the method of grouping a market into smaller subgroups – is the process of target marketing. Market segments can be geographic (as in a certain region or climate), demographic (by age or race), psychographic (concerning attitudes, behaviors, lifestyles, or loyalty characteristics), or historical (regarding previous customers).

For example, if the practice's services are confined to a specific geographic area, then the target market can be further defined to reflect the number of users of the service within that geographic segment. If an orthopedic practice in Aspen, Colo., is marketing its products and services, it will most likely target its efforts to the surrounding town – the local hospital, employers, ski companies, resorts, hotels, and lodges where injured skiers or family members may return to seek recommendations.

Once target markets are identified, the practice needs to develop a marketing mix that is positioned to be attractive to that segment. The marketing mix enables practices to join together different marketing decision areas, such as products, prices, promotions, and place – also known as the 4Ps – to develop an overall marketing plan.[42]

Products

In medical group practices, products are typically services; with regard to marketing mix and marketing plan development, these services should be used as marketing resources, and a focal point should be differentiation of the practice's services from that of the competition. For example, the orthopedic practice in Aspen may offer a product line that includes orthopedic consultation, radiology services, surgery, and possibly physical therapy or medical massage, in addition to medical equipment such as crutches, bandages, or braces.

Prices

Determining the total cost to the customer is part of the pricing element. Pricing decisions should take into account profit margins and the probable pricing response of competitors. How the practice prices its services is critical because it will have a direct effect on the success of the practice. Pricing strategies and computations can be complex, but the basic rules of pricing are straightforward:

- All prices must cover costs;
- The best and most effective way of lowering prices is to lower costs;
- Prices must reflect the dynamics of cost, demand, changes in the market, and response to competition;
- Prices must be established to ensure sales. Don't price against a competitive operation alone; rather, price to sell;
- Product utility, longevity, maintenance, and end use must be judged continually, and target prices adjusted accordingly; and
- Prices must be set to preserve order in the marketplace.[43]

Many methods of establishing prices are available to practices, among them:

- *Cost-plus pricing* is used mainly by manufacturers. This method assures that all costs, both fixed and variable, are covered and the desired profit percentage is attained.
- *Demand pricing* is used by practices that sell their services/products through a variety of sources at differing prices based on demand.
- *Competitive pricing* is used by practices that are entering a market where there is already an established price and it is difficult to differentiate one product from another.

- *Markup pricing* is used mainly by retailers and does not necessarily apply to medical practices. Markup pricing is calculated by adding the desired profit to the cost of the product.[44]

Promotion

Promotion decisions are those related to communicating and selling to potential customers and usually involve selling, sales promotions, advertising, and public relations – with only the latter two applicable to most group practices. A practice's use of promotion is accomplished through communications about the practice to potential customers. Again, think about the orthopedists in Aspen. For promotion they may choose to place their efforts on television or radio advertisements, listings in the phone book, announcements about the practice in the local newspaper, public service announcements, and community service programs.

Place

Place, meaning placement or distribution, refers to decisions regarding market coverage, member selection, logistics, levels of service, and convenience to the customer. Distribution decisions are best made by analyzing competitors to determine the channels they are using and then deciding whether to use the same type of channel or an alternative that may provide the practice with a strategic advantage. The distribution strategy chosen by the practice will also be based on factors in addition to the channels being used by its competition, including pricing strategy and internal resources. For example, perhaps the orthopedic practice's administrator finds that the competition runs advertising in the Saturday newspaper. S/he may choose to run placement of the practice's ad head-to-head on Saturday, or may decide to run the ad on Sunday, or use another, completely different media for advertising instead – for example, sponsoring the equipment for a local youth group's ski club or the prizes for a downhill race.

Positioning

Although not a part of E. Jerome McCarthy's original 4Ps of the marketing mix, there is a fifth P for practices to consider as well –

positioning. A practice's positioning strategy is affected by a number of variables that are closely tied to the motivations and requirements of target customers as well as the actions of primary competitors.

Before a product can be positioned, several strategic questions need to be addressed, such as: How are the practice's competitors positioning themselves (e.g., the region's best at shoulders, arms, and hand surgery)? What specific attributes do your practice's services have that its competitors do not (e.g., radiology in house)? What customer needs does the practice's service fulfill (e.g., emergency consultation)? Once these questions have been addressed based on market research, the practice executive can then begin to develop a positioning strategy illustrating exactly how it wants its services perceived by both customers and the competition.

Practice Structure and Culture

The marketing plan in general, as well as specific tasks such as the development of the marketing mix, should take into consideration the structure and culture of the practice. Structural features of the practice are formal, usually inflexible, created and maintained by documentation, and contingency-centered – they set responsibilities, formal rights, and rewards or punishments on which individual behavior or group action is contingent.[45] The structure determines how the practice is supposed to operate and for what purpose. The culture of the practice, in contrast, is informal, flexible, created and maintained by word of mouth, and ideology-centered: it defines good and bad, winning and losing, friends and enemies, and so forth.[46] The cultural characterizations of the practice – people, circumstances, events, objects, facts, processes, and information – are critical for practice decisions and progress. Structure and culture are unique to each practice and shape the image that the practice presents to the community.

The marketing plan for the practice should align with the practice's structure and culture, its style and image, and what makes the practice unique. "Truth in marketing/advertising" is an adage that applies well here. Marketing materials should accurately depict the practice, and the messages utilized should be shared by members of the practice. For example, if the practice has a culture of building relationships with patients, the marketing materials should reflect this, rather than focus on maintaining high efficiency and quick turnaround in seeing patients. The style or image of the practice must be evaluated.

Advertising

The final component of the marketing plan addresses advertising, which relates to the topic of promotion previously discussed. Gone are the days when a practice could "hang out a shingle" and the phone would begin to ring. Health care is an extremely competitive marketplace that requires practices to often rely on innovative advertising practices. Today's practices are, in every sense of the word, "businesses," and they must utilize advertising concepts that were once shunned by the health care industry, such as direct-to-consumer marketing through television and radio advertisements, direct mail, public seminars, creation of Internet Websites or newsletters, and even use of billboards or other signage. The choice of advertising method should be guided by consideration of the following questions:

- What is the source of the practice's current patients?
- What method is optimal for conveying the practice's "message"?
- What method will reach the largest concentration of potential customers?
- What is the cost per unit (i.e., new patient) for this type of method? What is the expected return on investment?
- Is this method ethical in all possible respects?

Once an advertising method has been selected, the practice needs to ensure that the materials designed are written at an appropriate reading level and are clear, concise, and appealing, taking into consideration the population most likely to be served by the practice. Advertising materials, as with all other components of the marketing plan, also need to accurately and honestly portray the practice.

■ Summary

It is no longer effective to identify target customers and then try to let them know how good the practice is or that the practice wants their business. Instead, the practice must be able to differentiate itself in terms of how it recruits and trains, how it manages people and work, how it uses technology to add value to the customer (in addition to the ways the competition uses it), what new services or products it is offering, how it advertises and promotes these products and services, and more. A marketing plan will assist the practice in accomplishing these goals.

TASK 4 **Monitor and Evaluate Effectiveness of Strategic, Business, and Marketing Plan Activities**

EACH OF THE PLANNING DOCUMENTS should specify who is responsible for the overall implementation of the plan as well as who is responsible for achieving each goal and objective. The plans should also specify who is responsible for monitoring the implementation of the plans and making decisions based on the results. For example, a board might expect the practice executive to regularly report to the full board about the status of implementation, including progress toward each of the overall strategic goals. In turn, the practice executive might expect regular status reports from department heads or clinical staff regarding the status toward their achieving the goals and objectives assigned to them.

■ Monitoring and Evaluation

What Is Monitoring?

Monitoring is a procedure for checking the effectiveness and efficiency in implementing a plan by identifying strengths and shortcomings and recommending corrective measures to optimize the intended outcomes. In the monitoring process, plan execution performance is compared against parameters defined in a baseline plan, and corrective actions are taken, where necessary, in seeking to implement the plan within the constraints of defined time, cost, and quality parameters.

Monitoring provides the basis for minimizing or preventing schedule and cost overruns while ensuring that required quality standards are achieved in the implementation stage of the plans. Among the numerous benefits of monitoring are that it:

- Identifies flaws in the design and execution plans;
- Recommends changes to the practice's implementation plans;
- Establishes whether the goals, objectives, and strategies are carried out according to the plans;
- Continually reviews the plans' assumptions, thereby assessing the risk;
- Establishes the likelihood of output achievement as planned;
- Verifies that plan outputs continue to support the project purpose;
- Establishes links between the performance of operations in progress and future needs and requirements;
- Identifies recurrent problems that need attention and helps identify solutions;
- Identifies supplements to plans required to enhance their effectiveness;
- Provides a basis for projecting the completion schedule and costs based on current performance; and
- Identifies the situations necessary for activating contingency plans.[47]

What Is Evaluation?

Evaluation involves the application of rigorous methods to assess the extent to which plans have achieved their defined objectives. It is a process that attempts to determine, as systematically and objectively as possible, the relevance, effectiveness, efficiency, and impact (both intentional and unintentional) of the plans in the context of their stated objectives.

Evaluating each of the practice's plans will generate information to help practice executives:

- Improve the economic performance of new and ongoing services and strategies;

- Choose among various development alternatives;

- Learn about best practices in a given field;

- Determine the extent to which the project justification was achieved;

- Enhance the sustainability of the practice's deliverables; and

- Make decisions on the identification and implementation of supplementary and complementary services.[48]

Key Components

In the monitoring and evaluation stage, there are a few key components that, when present, assist in the success of this stage of the plan(s). For example, a timetable helps to determine whether implementation is on schedule. It also helps to identify what tasks are on schedule in comparison to those that are not. Another key component is a good record-keeping system, which enables the practice executive to monitor the impact of the plan(s) and to make necessary adjustments to ensure success. As past results are studied and compared to preselected guidelines, any changes from expected results can provide an early warning system for potential problems. For records to be useful, they must be properly summarized, analyzed, and thoroughly studied. External trends and events that may provide additional opportunities or pose threats to the practice's plan should also be continually monitored. Finally, it is important for the practice to understand that, in most cases, it is not possible at the onset to completely design an evaluation plan that will do exactly what the practice wants it to do. More realistically, such a plan unfolds as succeeding phases of the evaluation process are carried out. Continuous revision of plans is normally done as each step evolves. This need for revision, however, is not meant to underestimate the importance of a master plan that will provide initial and overall guidance during the process.[49]

Key Questions to Ask

In the monitoring and evaluation stages of the planning process, several key questions should be asked by the medical practice executive to ensure that each of the plans is on target. The most important question to ask is: Are goals and objectives being achieved? If they are, the practice executive should then recognize, reward, and communicate the progress. If not, s/he should consider the following questions:

- Will the goals be achieved according to the time lines specified in the plan? If not, why not?

- Should the deadlines for completion be changed? (The practice manager should be careful about making these time changes before determining why efforts are behind schedule.)

- Have adequate resources (money, equipment, facilities, training, and so forth) been allocated to allow staff to achieve the goals?

- Are the goals and objectives still realistic?

- Should priorities be changed to put more focus on achieving the goals?

- Should the goals be changed? (The practice manager should also be careful about making these changes before determining why efforts are not achieving the goals.)

- What can be learned from monitoring and evaluation to improve future planning activities and also to improve future monitoring and evaluation efforts?[50]

Steps in Plan Monitoring and Evaluation

There are three essential activities in monitoring and evaluating a medical practice's plans. The first is identifying and defining the

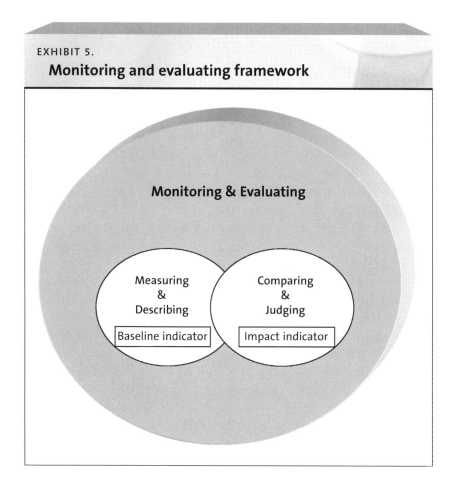

EXHIBIT 5.

Monitoring and evaluating framework

attributes of baseline indicators. For example, if the practice were to use patient satisfaction rates to indicate practice quality in a new service, the measure of the current level of satisfaction (before commencement of the new service) would be a baseline indicator. The second activity is defining the planned level of performance, which is usually denominated in terms of a planned satisfaction rate of 95 percent by a stated date. This rate implies that the success of the new service will be measured by the extent to which it has achieved this level of patient satisfaction. This is an impact indicator. The final activity involves evaluating the performance of the practice.

The practice will state how it intends to measure performance to determine the level of satisfaction achieved. This evaluation may require conducting a survey some years after the implementation of the new service, when the impact of the new service may be measurable. This process is known as evaluation.[51]

These three activities can be further delineated into a monitoring and evaluation process that utilizes two primary sets of elements: (1) measuring and describing, and (2) comparing and judging (see Exhibit 5). In this framework, measuring is the process of determining or describing whether there has been a change in the variables that may have been manipulated (e.g., the addition of new services by the practice). Using the above example, the practice decides whether the new service it provided caused the change that was expected in the form of an objective or standard. Did the practice improve patient satisfaction by providing a new service? In the measuring process, quantifiable terms are used to describe what has actually happened.

Comparison is an important component because it allows the practice to compare *what is* (at some point after the service has been established or some defined time line) with *what was* (prior to the service being provided). Similarly, the idea of an evaluation model may be to compare *what is* with *what should be* as established by the practice's plans, by the practice's expectations, and by the practice's original objectives. The key is that the practice compares progress (what actually happened) to a standard that it, as an agent of change, had originally established. Did the practice improve patient satisfaction by 10 percent as it set out to do? To what extent were the objectives met?[52]

The evaluator's judgment becomes very important at this point. It involves a decision(s) relative to the extent that the differences between the comparisons are important. These differences, or variances, should stimulate questions: Why did one decision cost more (or less)? Were objectives met? Is a positive variance a cost saving or a failure to implement? Is a negative variance a change in plans, a management failure, or an unrealistic budget? In answering these questions, judgment may involve the practice's experiences, knowledge accumulated, and the ability to see relationships objectively.

Ultimately, the practice executive will decide whether a course of action led to an outcome that was useful.[53]

Monitoring and Evaluation Frameworks

Three basic frameworks are often used in monitoring- and evaluation-related activities:

1. Benchmark/indicator guidelines, introduced at the project preparation (or design) stage;

2. A framework incorporating the concepts of continued rationale, efficiency, effectiveness, effects and lessons learned, used during implementation and completion and after the completion stages for evaluations; and

3. A framework featuring areas of summative evaluation (strategy, policy, design, monitoring and execution, procedures, performance, sustainability) used for impact evaluation.[54]

Systems Design for a Monitoring and Evaluation System

Monitoring and evaluation of each of the plans should be integrated within and across the practice. Several off-the-shelf software packages that facilitate the processes of planning, execution, controlling, monitoring, evaluation, and reporting may be useful in this integration, including MindManager™, Microsoft® Project™, and the Balanced Scorecard™ system.

MindManager is a software tool for brainstorming and planning that enables planning teams within practices to design clear, well-planned documents at the beginning of the plan. MindManager is based on a visual mapping of ideas, knowledge, and information. It enables users to quickly and efficiently capture ideas generated from team brainstorming, identify user requirements, classify risk areas, and recognize stakeholder issues. MindManager is also able to plan scope, assign tasks and time lines, and when necessary, export this information to Microsoft Project for use in project planning.

Microsoft Project is a powerful planning and monitoring software tool used in developing plan schedules, assigning resources to tasks, and developing the plan budget. It has the capability to consolidate logically related projects to show information at the practice level, and provides a basis for showing plan execution performance against the baseline plan.

The *Balanced Scorecard* system is a strategic management approach that translates a vision into a clear set of objectives or critical success factors. Key performance indicators measure each objective's performance, representing a broad range of outcome measures and performance drivers. It allows the analysis of the cause and effect of processes needed to successfully implement strategies with built-in measurements to track progress. The Balanced Scorecard system emphasizes leading indicators of future performance along with the tracking of past performance, which are often stated in financial terms.

Frequency of Monitoring and Evaluation

The frequency of reviews depends on the nature of the practice and the environment in which it is operating. Practices experiencing rapid change from inside and/or outside the practice may want to monitor implementation of the plan at least on a monthly basis. Boards of directors should see the status of implementation at least on a quarterly basis. Practice executives should see the status at least on a monthly basis.

Reporting Results of Monitoring and Evaluation

Ideally, the process of monitoring and evaluating the implementation of the plans would include three key elements: internal progress report, external review, and an annual "report card."

Internal Progress Report

Internally, a key to monitoring and evaluating the progress of the plan(s) would be regular progress reports completed by the practice staff assigned to each goal or strategy. The completion of these progress reports should be timed to be compatible with the practice's annual budget cycle. The progress reports would describe the actions taken by the practice toward achieving specific outcomes and strategies of each of the plans, and might include costs, benefits, performance measures, and progress to date. The progress reports should be online documents to facilitate the ease with which they are submitted for review. The board and practice executive should review the progress reports and serve as the overall internal monitors for the plans.

External Review

Externally, an independent review committee could assist with monitoring and providing feedback on the practice's progress in implementing the plans, much in the same way as external stakeholders may provide oversight to the planning processes. The review committee might be made up of consumers (e.g., current patients) and other stakeholders from diverse backgrounds. This external committee should meet at least annually to review progress reports from the practice. The committee could review and comment on the semi-annual reports, and forward its feedback to the practice.

Report Cards

At the end of each year, an annual "report card" should be produced. This annual report card would evaluate the year's activities related to each of the plans based upon how well the practice has furthered the achievement of the outcomes and strategies of the plans. The practice report card also can serve as a benchmarking tool. The outcomes and results for the practice can be compared to local, regional, and national figures to give a complete picture of the practice's achievements.

Report Content and Feedback

Each of these reports – internal, external, and report card – should describe answers to the key questions while monitoring implementation; trends regarding the progress (or lack thereof) toward specific goals and objectives; recommendations about the status; and any actions needed to be taken by the practice.[55]

A mechanism to receive feedback from the recipients of each of these reports – such as a mailed questionnaire or survey, a follow-up telephone call, or adding an agenda item for discussion of the plans at a meeting – is another important consideration. Once the shareholders involved have the opportunity to analyze the materials sent to them, they will often have comments, concerns, or additional information that the practice probably will want to assess. It is imperative that systems be in place to allow this type of consensus building and follow-up.

Plan Modification: Deviating from or Changing the Plans

It is acceptable, and at times even expected, to deviate from the plan. The plan is only a guideline, not a strict road map that must be followed. The practice changes its direction somewhat as it proceeds through the coming years. Changes in the plan usually result from changes in the practice's external environment; changes in customer needs, resulting in different practice goals; and/or changes in the availability of resources to carry out the original plan, etc. In addition, feedback can demonstrate that shareholders have expressed concerns not otherwise considered. The most important aspect of deviating from the plan is understanding why the deviation is necessary (e.g., having a solid understanding of what is going on and why).

The practice should also ensure that it has a mechanism identified for changing the plans, if necessary. This mechanism should address what is causing changes to be made; why the changes should be made; and what changes are to be made, including to goals, objectives, responsibilities, and time lines. When changes are made to plans, the practice should document what can be learned from recent planning activities to make the next planning activities more efficient.

Planning is a cyclical process that involves numerous checks and balances. Continuous education of physicians and practice staff in the many steps involved in the planning cycle, and consensus building among all involved in the planning process, are crucial in the practice's planning success.

■ Summary

If the evaluation process is to contribute to performance, the practice manager must assure the practice and its stakeholders that the evaluation is impartial, credible, useful, participatory, provides feedback, and is cost-beneficial.[56] Even though evaluating and monitoring each of the plans does not guarantee success, potential problems may be averted by using a formalized method of evaluation. Additionally, such a method provides an opportunity for the practice to make adjustments before major problems arise.

TASK 5 **Pursue and Establish Partnerships and Strategic Alliances**

THE BENEFITS OF ALLIANCES are undeniable. According to Ernst and Young, organizations that form successful alliances can earn more than 20 percent of their revenues in such relationships.[57] In fact, this number has grown and continues to increase. Research indicates that some organizations expect their alliances to contribute 35 percent of their revenues in the future, up from 21 percent in 1998 and 15 percent in 1995.[58]

An alliance is a cooperative arrangement between two or more physician groups that allows these organizations to combine in a common effort to gain or maintain competitive advantage. The mere formation of an alliance does not guarantee success, but rather requires mutual participation of all parties, a viable business concept, and a realistic strategy to implementing that idea.[59]

Alliances should be strategic in nature rather than a short-term solution to an immediate problem. Medical practice executives need to look past short-term gains and focus on building long-term goals for alliances and partnerships.

■ Key Issues in Alliances

A number of key questions should be considered when forming an alliance, including:

- What is the purpose of the alliance?
- What partner or partners should be selected?
- What is the structure of the alliance?
- What are the roles and responsibilities of the parties involved?
- What are the risks involved?
- What is the duration of the alliance?

Purpose of the Alliance

Prior to considering an alliance, a clearly defined purpose has to be established. Without a clear vision, organizations will waste time, money, and energy entering into alliances and partnerships that do not meet their organization's needs.

The primary motivation for many health care organizations to engage in alliances and partnerships is due to the conflicting demands of cost-containment, delivering high-quality care, and expanding access to services. Alliances and partnerships are the vehicles that enable medical group practices that do not possess the necessary resources individually to combine resources with other organizations to gain competitive advantage in the health care marketplace.[60]

Competitive advantage typically serves two purposes: (1) reduce dependence, and (2) improve organizational capacity. Ways in which organizations reduce dependence can be achieved through vertical integration, by which individual practices provide complementary services, thereby expanding access to a wider variety of services for their patients. By forming alliances, an individual organization is able to gain access to technology, expertise, labor, and possibly even capital, thus expanding its capacity. Another way practices can increase organizational capacity is by forming alliances to share risk, so that individual organizations can enter new markets without having to bear all the financial risk of uncertain conditions inherent in new ventures. Alliances also help individual organizations to overcome regulatory barriers, increase organizational flexibility, improve access to technological innovations, and achieve efficiency through economies of scale.[61]

Partner Selection

It is critical to select alliance partners that leverage one another's strengths. Alliances are not a quick fix for all of an organization's deficiencies. Alliances are similar to relationships – each person has a distinct identity and personality. Alliances, like relationships, unite unique parties to work together for a common cause. Just like relationships, however, there are negatives associated with alliances as well. Alliances bring organizations' employees together, with any cultural differences they may have. For instance, one organization may possess formal, clear management structures, while the other operates informally and forms only ad hoc arrangements. To be successful, alliance partners must share compatible, but not necessarily identical, cultures and missions or the alliance will fail.

Differences can be a source of conflict, and they should be anticipated. Alliance partners need to keep their common interests in mind at all times. The following tips can help to resolve most conflicts that arise in alliances: (1) clarify the issue; (2) have each organization present its point of view; (3) seek to understand each partner's point of view; (4) discuss differences that arise; and (5) always agree to solve the problem collaboratively.[62]

It is the medical practice executive's role to watch for these warning signs of conflict and in a productive way to resolve it.[63] Warning signs that conflict is imminent include: (1) an issue repeatedly arises, (2) individual(s) choose not to listen during meetings and discussions, and (3) individuals seem to avoid one another. Practice executives should be proactive to overcome possible shortcomings before they become a major issue.

This initial step in establishing an alliance requires screening and selecting potential partners. In order to do so, it is critical first to understand the practice's own objectives, its capabilities, and its resources or lack thereof. Without a full understanding and accounting for all alliance strategy issues internally, decisions about whom to partner with will be uninformed.[64]

Ideal candidates for alliances will have compatible objectives, complementary resources and skills, an organizational fit in terms of culture and processes, and a willingness to ally with each other. Although collecting this information can be difficult and time consuming, the payoff for understanding a potential partner's objectives, financials, resources, skills, processes, and culture can be priceless.[65] It is also important to consult with each potential practice's legal counsel to understand the ramifications of aligning with a particular organization.

Choosing the Appropriate Structure

When considering alliances, many models are available to strengthen a practice's competitive position. Depending on the level of integration or degree of cooperation required, organizations can pick from any of the following types of affiliations. In general, this list begins with the least integrated and finishes with the most complex.

Network Affiliation

Network affiliations are the least-integrated type of alliance and function as a club with a general purpose. They provide a useful avenue for supportive dialogue, communication, and commiseration; however, they are not functional for contracting or for implementation activities.[66]

Joint Ventures

Joint ventures are typically formed for a well-defined goal that is typically focused on capital projects. According to Ginter, Swayne, and Duncan, "a joint venture is the combination of the resources of two or more separate organizations to accomplish a designated task....When projects get too large, technology too expensive, or the costs of failure too high for a single organization, joint ventures are often used."[67] The term "joint venture" applies to a wide range of interorganizational arrangements and frequently concerns physician-related ventures.

Joint ventures can provide medical practices with a competitive strategy, typically in an undeveloped or underdeveloped market, moving more directly from existing providers to a more convenient alternative for a targeted population. One advantage of joint ventures is that they can be quickly formed to take advantage of fast-moving opportunities. They also allow organizations otherwise constrained by resources and capabilities to effectively pursue opportunities together.[68]

As in all the models of alliances, joint ventures can be difficult due to the clash of culture and compatibility between organizations. Allied organizations need to be on the same page, but need not abandon their identity or their organizational culture to collaborate successfully. To avoid casualties from the culture clash, explicit mechanisms need to be developed to identify and manage these challenges.[69]

Independent Provider Associations (IPAs) and Provider Organizations (POs)

IPAs and POs are typically formed to organize independent medical group practices for the purpose of contracting with health maintenance organizations (HMOs) and purchasing supplies or other services. The main difference between IPAs and POs is that IPAs typically are affiliated with a hospital.[70]

One primary advantage of IPAs is that they offer a variety of physician choices to their members. They also tend to be more acceptable to managed care organizations (MCOs) than other, less traditional integrated delivery system models. Another reason IPAs are attractive is that they require much less capital to start and maintain as opposed to other models available.[71]

IPAs are not without disadvantages, though. For example, because IPAs are one of the least-integrated forms of alliances, they do not offer the opportunity to leverage resources and achieve economies of scale that more integrated forms offer. In addition, management of this loose type of alliance structure can be challenging because individual physician practices maintain their independence in an IPA. This issue grows as more practices enter the IPA.[72]

Physician/Hospital Organizations (PHOs)

PHOs involve physicians and hospitals whereby they become partners in the delivery of health care. Exclusivity is an issue because most PHOs contain a selection process to qualify the doctors involved. The ownership arrangements of PHOs vary widely; however, most strive to provide physicians and hospitals an equal voice and ownership. In most PHOs, the hospital organization may supply the most capital; however, board composition does not typically reflect this equity position.[73]

PHOs have the advantage of being inexpensive to form and maintain. They are also desirable to many group practices because they maintain group autonomy and, thus, are nonthreatening. One of the biggest advantages that PHOs provide is the ability to negotiate on behalf of their membership. Additionally, they provide an opportunity for greater integration between a hospital and its medical staff.[74]

Along with these advantages come several disadvantages, including the unpredictable nature of these affiliations. Because these affiliations are loose, they are often ineffective and do not provide partners with economies of scale or improvement in contracting ability. In fact, MCOs often view PHOs as a barrier to effective communication with individual practitioners, thus decreasing the effectiveness of utilization of management activities.[75] MCOs often choose to deal directly with individual physicians because they desire the right to select providers themselves.

Management Services Organizations (MSOs)

MSOs are typically formed to provide management services and administrative systems to one or more medical group practices. MSOs are normally based on one or more health care organizations. For example, MSOs may conduct billing, marketing, or perhaps the human resource functions for its members. Each medical practice remains a separate entity and chooses whether to use the services that the MSO offers. In addition to providing the above services, many MSOs purchase the assets of the physicians' practice.[76]

MSOs are more closely aligned with the hospital as compared to PHOs. MSOs provide their members the economies of scale and also the advantage of sharing data regarding practice behavior, which can help to increase the effectiveness of individual practices.[77]

Similar to the PHO, physicians in an MSO remain independent contractors and thus maintain the ability to change allegiances, a downside to this type of affiliation. This point may also be considered an advantage, though, especially from the physician's viewpoint. Another disadvantage is the hospital mind-set, in which physician practices are viewed as another hospital department, negatively impacting the practice's performance.[78]

Group Practice without Walls (GPWW)

GPWWs are not true alliances because individual groups or sites can continue to manage themselves. GPWWs offer a higher level of integration of physician services and do not require the participation of a hospital organization. Most GPWWs are formed to address antitrust or hazards of the Stark self-referral law. In fact, a GPWW is a legal merging of all assets of the physician practice, which is different than the acquisition of tangible assets, as in the MSO.[79]

An advantage of this type of affiliation is that each site maintains its independence, and thus is easy to manage and does not have to sacrifice much autonomy; however, GPWWs help to present a united front to MCOs because they have the legal ability to negotiate and commit resources on behalf of their members. Due to the increased level of integration, GPWWs are able to achieve a moderate level of economies of scale. Examples may include shared billing, group purchasing, contracting for human resources, and payroll. Because the financial performances of its members are dependent upon one another, GPWWs are able to exert pressure and influence the practice behavior of their members.[80]

Perhaps the primary disadvantage associated with GPWWs is the fact that individual medical practices are still independent. This can present a managerial challenge to align incentives, even though fiscal performance in a GPWW is dependent on one another. Another disadvantage that is linked to the independence of the physician practices is that the overall leadership is typically weaker than that found in the medical groups that form the GPWW.[81]

Single-Specialty Group Practices

Single-specialty group practices include only physicians of the same specialty and provide a significant level of integration. Single-specialty groups share a common billing number, fee schedule, benefits package, and a formal governance structure.

Multispecialty Group Practices

Multispecialty group practices are group practices that include multiple specialties and disciplines. Multispecialty group practices must be formed to ensure that the group includes the right mix of specialties and the appropriate proportions to allow for a mutually beneficial existence.[82]

Multispecialty group practices are advantageous because they can accept capitation, are able to leverage economies of scale, offer an environment conducive for the exchange of ideas between physicians, and are attractive to MCOs. Despite these advantages, they have the potential to threaten the existing autonomy of individual specialties and consequently can be functionally challenging to manage.[83]

Due Diligence Process

To minimize exposure to risk when embarking on a strategic alliance or partnership, it is critical to conduct due diligence to ensure that the proposed venture is a prudent decision. Due diligence entails collecting information and data in order to assess the feasibility of a particular venture so that a decision is reached only after considering all prudent viewpoints. Due diligence should take place on numerous fronts, including recruiting, membership in a strategic alliance, considering managed care contracts, adopting new technology, marketing campaigns, and compensation of employees. Due diligence is a complex activity, especially in light of considering strategic alliances. Thus, a knowledgeable health care attorney should be consulted when considering opportunities and drafting essential legal documents.[84]

Recruiting

Ensuring the effective and successful recruitment of personnel, including physicians, is a critical responsibility of the medical practice executive. Due diligence should be conducted to ensure that personnel are qualified and that they fit the culture of the organization. Medical practice executives should understand the marketplace prior to conducting a search process so they can respond to candidates' questions, be familiar with the most effective sources for personnel, set clear expectations about the time frame needed for the search, and understand the financial implications of attracting and hiring staff.[85]

In addition, medical practices need to present an appealing practice environment in order to attract quality personnel. Prospective employees are not only interested in pleasant surroundings, they are also concerned with the financial stability, up-to-date technology, and attractive schedules and policies. By ensuring that these concerns are addressed, medical practice executives will be more successful in selling the organization to prospective employees and reduce failure and future turnover.[86]

Due diligence is especially critical when recruiting physicians to join the medical practice. If due diligence is not practiced, effective personnel will not be attracted or retained, and thus the organization will likely perform poorly or fail.

Strategic Alliances

Due diligence is a crucial part of the alliance process. Thus, whenever feasible, a more comprehensive due diligence investigation should be undertaken when considering whether to partner with a particular organization. However, due to the costly and time-consuming nature of the process, it is not always feasible to investigate every detail of a potential strategic alliance. Thus, when considering smaller alliances and transactions, too much due diligence can kill the transaction.[87]

Key questions to assist in the due diligence of a potential strategic alliance include the following:

- What in the alliance is important to your medical group practice? What isn't?

- Which problems will be costly? Which ones will be minor?
- Where are you likely to find problems? Where are you unlikely to find problems?
- What type of transaction are you expecting? How large or small is the transaction? How complex? What will the due diligence investigation cost in time and money?
- What is the risk to your medical group practice if the unexpected causes the transaction to go bad?
- How much time do you have? What do you have to lose by delay? What does the potential partner have to lose? How important to your medical practice is the alliance? How important is your practice to the potential partners?[88]

Additionally, more specific questions can be asked to further clarify whether a potential merger is a prudent move. For instance:

- What is the organization's public image? Have there been any tensions between the community and the organization?
- Are there any pending lawsuits against the organization?
- Does the organization have a good reputation?
- How long has the organization been in business?
- Is the organization financially stable?[89]

Managed Care Contracts

When considering partnerships and strategic alliances, it is critical to review all managed care contracts – both old and new. Frequently, new alliances may change the structure of current contracts, particularly the reimbursement mechanisms for physicians. Thus, it is important to review and decide whether to continue the contracts in the present form or make changes. Another important consideration regarding managed care contracting is that the structure of the proposed partnership or alliance may actually make renegotiating contracts more favorable for reimbursement levels.[90]

Technology

The technological know-how of each partner involved in a potential alliance must also be considered due to the costly nature of technology. For instance, if the medical practice is currently using a paper-based medical records system, it may be inordinately expensive to convert to electronic health records to facilitate the alliance. Often, the expense of adopting new technology may outweigh the benefits of the potential partnership.

Marketing

The power of marketing cannot be overlooked. A carefully constructed marketing campaign can assist a new partnership or alliance in rapidly succeeding, especially in generating cash flow. Thus, medical practice executives need to carefully align marketing to showcase their new organizational form to make the practice's current patients, future patients, and the medical community aware of its existence to retain or expand its current client base.[91]

Physician Compensation

Physician compensation must be carefully evaluated prior to considering potential partnerships and alliances. Conflict can arise when a medical practice whose physicians are dependent upon a salary compensation structure attempt to partner or align with a practice whose physicians have an ownership approach to compensation. Another area to consider is that of benefits packages, as physicians in integrated organizations typically receive more generous packages than a new group can offer, thus potentially contributing to discord.[92]

Roles and Responsibilities

Successful alliances require well-defined processes to address key issues in alliance formation, implementation, and operation; thus, it is necessary to structure and negotiate agreement with each partner. The strategic objectives of the alliance should be evaluated and aligned to increase the probability of success. It is at this stage that staffing decisions should be considered, with all partners striving for a reasonable share of control that facilitates equitable involvement from all sides. Because alliances are a long-term venture, it is advisable to commit the best personnel who are striving for long-term placement; otherwise, high turnover can doom the alliance before it gets started. Alliance relationships take time to build and gain trust; thus frequently changing alliance personnel can disrupt the process.[93] Knowledge about the practice's capabilities is particularly important for defining work roles and supporting the requirements of current and future partners.[94]

At the outset of the partnership, alliance partners should collaboratively set goals and measure performance parameters that are quantifiable. These goals and measures should be congruent with the alliance's primary objectives. Additionally, alliance partners should address governance issues and develop an operating framework built around the clearly defined roles and expectations of each partner. Without resolving these critical issues, the success of the alliance may be in jeopardy.

Risks

Risk is a significant factor in the formation of alliances because strategic decision making is ultimately concerned with assessing odds for success.[95] One of the primary advantages of joining an alliance is to control uncertainty and exposure to risk. Risk can be defined as unanticipated or negative variation, typically associated with negative outcomes. Risk sharing or risk controlling is a key justification for joining strategic alliances.[96]

Two types of risks are generally associated with alliances: (1) relational risk, or the probability that one or more partners does not comply with the rules governing the alliance; and (2) performance risk, which refers to the probability that the intended strategic goals of the alliance may not be achieved despite diligent cooperation among the partners.[97]

Duration

Just as strategic plans, alliances should be reviewed and evaluated on an annual basis to estimate their effectiveness and worth – similar to how a portfolio of investments should be viewed. Using this approach allows the organizations to manage, review, and evaluate alliances as an aggregate business, and it permits the organization to evaluate current resource allocations with a focus on identifying how alliance concentrations contribute to possible duplication or gaps.[98]

While conducting an ongoing evaluation, it is important for the organization to develop an effective working environment with all partners to facilitate the completion of the actual work. It is critical to include performance measures combined with feedback from alliance partners to assess the progress of the alliance.

If an alliance is not functioning as intended and is not salvageable, it is appropriate to end the association. Often, this is due to a change in market conditions, and no one is to blame for the ending of the alliance. Regardless of the reason for the termination of the alliance, it is important for the practice to maintain a positive relationship with the former partners, as new opportunities for collaboration will present themselves in the future.[99]

■ Managing Partnerships and Strategic Alliances

Management of alliances should be approached in a fashion similar to how organizations should be managed. As in all organizations, medical practice executives should continually acknowledge and actively monitor the concerns of all legitimate stakeholders and shareholders, and should take their interests into consideration when making operational decisions. A stakeholder is anyone who has an investment in the success of the organization, including physicians, administrators, patients, vendors, and the community. Shareowners have a special status among stakeholders in that the potential gain or loss from their involvement with the corporation is determined by the organization's profit margin.[100]

Practice executives should maintain open lines of communication with stakeholders about their respective concerns and contributions, and about the risks that they assume due to their involvement with the corporation.[101] The more open managers can be about critical decisions and their consequences, and the more clearly managers understand and appreciate the perspectives and concerns of affected parties, the more likely it is that problematic situations can be satisfactorily resolved. Open communication and dialogue are, in themselves, stakeholder benefits, quite apart from their content or the conclusions.[102]

By virtue of being part of an alliance, organizations lose some freedom to make decisions without concern for alliance partners. The medical practice executive should be sensitive to the concerns and capabilities of the other alliance stakeholders. To maintain the survival of the alliance, the interdependence of efforts among the alliance partners must be recognized. All attempts should be made to achieve a fair distribution of rewards and burdens in the alliance, and at the same time to account for each organization's vulnerabilities.[103]

A commitment to engage in dialogue, however, does not constitute a commitment to collective decision making. There are obvious limits to the amount and content of information (particularly information about strategic options under consideration) that can be appropriately shared with particular stakeholder groups.

Practice executives should acknowledge that conflict is an inevitable part of alliances, as it is with all interactions with people. In the interests of all parties involved, any conflicts should be handled openly and fairly, and, where necessary, by third-party review. Maintaining fairness and openness will guarantee that all parties will act responsibly and not threaten the existence of the alliance.[104]

■ Conclusion

An appreciation of alliances can assist medical practice executives in understanding the resources and dedication necessary to establish such partnerships. Alliances enable medical practices to strategically position themselves and gain competitive advantage to survive in today's turbulent health care market.

TASK 6 **Develop and Implement Community Outreach, Public Relations, and Customer Relations Programs**

DEVELOPING COMMUNITY OUTREACH, public relations, and customer relations programs is unique because these tasks are intangible. When designing such programs, the medical practice must take into account the aesthetics and psychological benefits to the target audience. To develop appropriate plans and programs, the practice must first define the community in which it operates. By definition, a community is a group of people who share a particular situation, whether that situation is living in the same area, going to the same house of worship, or another defining group. Being part of a community induces a duty to one another. Medical practices have a duty to provide residents in their geographic area with the best-quality health care.

■ Patient Education

Patient education is an important part of a medical practice's community outreach that also helps in maintaining practice visibility. Brochures, newsletters, videos, and medical practice Websites are common methods for patient education. The quality and content of these materials must be considered to ensure that the practice's aims and positioning goals are accomplished. In addition, due to the advances of technology and communication, there is a wider range of media from which to communicate with patients.

Patient Handbooks

A simple method for patient communication is the use of patient handbooks. These handbooks can be easily printed in-house due to the advances in personal computers and software, or they can be purchased through vendors. The purpose of a patient handbook is to communicate important information to help patients and their families better understand the treatment and care process. Patient handbooks enable patients and their families to play essential roles in the treatment of disease.

Patient-Communication Protocols

Communication is of the utmost importance in treating patients and their illnesses. Often, during the course of medical treatment, patients and their families are thrust into new and confusing experiences. It is the duty of physicians to ensure that all patient communications are clear and effective.

Verbal communication is the primary method used to convey health information to patients about their diagnosis and treatment options; however, verbal communication is fraught with difficulty. Supplementing verbal communication with written information and instruction is an essential part of establishing effective patient-communication protocols. Written material affords a patient the opportunity to read and reflect upon information when opportune, not just when s/he consults with the physician. Written brochures are usually readily available from professional associations as well as online.[105]

Medical practice executives should clearly outline patient-communication protocols so that all patients will receive the information necessary to make informed treatment decisions. Protocols should establish step-by-step instructions and include methods to assess patient understanding of physician instructions. Use of effective communication protocols will ensure that patients are informed; thus, such procedures can also be an effective risk management strategy.

Leveraging Technology

The Internet and other advances in technology have enabled even the smallest medical practices to engage in the practice of telehealth. Telehealth, like telemedicine, uses technology to provide clinical and medical services over geographic distances, rather than by traditional face-to-face methods, in a timely and convenient manner. In addition, telehealth also uses technology to deliver nonclinical medical services, such as patient education and administrative functions.[106]

Telehealth typically employs the use of interactive video to treat and interact with patients. Other telehealth methods include online discussion forums for the purpose of consultations and the ongoing management of patients. Telehealth can also provide patients and clinical professionals with education and training opportunities.[107]

Brochures

Brochures can be an effective method of educating patients about illnesses and courses of treatment; however, they can be expensive to purchase and time consuming to develop. On the positive side, brochures provide a written summary of what the patient needs to know about a particular procedure or condition. Studies have shown that informed patients are more likely to have better outcomes and require less staff time and attention.

An alternative to the printed brochure is to provide information via a medical practice Web page. Downloadable files can be used to transmit important information. An added advantage is the savings in printing costs, as well as the ability to update materials with little or no expense.

■ Community Focus/Collaboration

To be successful in today's health care environment, medical practices should have a defined strategy for interacting with the community. An organization's reputation, profitability, and even its continued existence can depend on the degree to which the community supports its efforts. By virtue of being health care providers, medical practices have an obligation to serve their communities. Therefore, it is critical for the medical practice executive to formulate a strategy to develop and maintain a community focus.

Awareness Building

One duty of medical practices is to build awareness of health issues impacting citizens. By virtue of collaborating with the community – both the citizenry and perhaps other medical practices – medical practices are able to actively involve those directly affected by certain issues. Collaboration in health initiatives enables co-learning, by which the community and medical practice contribute equally, and are thus able to achieve more than they would be able to do individually. Together, the partnership creates something new and valuable, thus creating a deeper commitment on behalf of all parties. Community collaborations help to "develop and maintain mutually respectful and dynamic partnerships with communities."[108]

Targeted Messages

Through the partnership synergy that results from deeply valuing one another's beliefs and knowledge, and through working in partnership with community residents, collaboration can help uncover the true needs of a community. Once these needs are identified, targeted messages can be developed to address any health problems that may exist. In addition, targeted health services can be developed to meet these needs as well.[109]

Cultural Sensitivity

Community collaboration can improve cultural sensitivity by virtue of working with disparate and diverse groups of people. When individuals come together to work on community problems, such as health problems, they learn to value the contributions of others, and hence to trust one another. In addition, individuals learn to value the differing perspectives that they previously did not. The value of the experiences obtained in collaborative work cannot be underestimated.

These experiences can help contribute to the cultural competency of the organization. By learning, understanding, and valuing cultural differences, practice patterns can be adjusted or reframed, so that treatment and health information can be delivered in a culturally acceptable manner.

Community Involvement

Community involvement is closely aligned with the mission of health care – to serve and help others. Thus, it is logical that individuals involved in health care would actively seek to participate in community activities and functions. Aside from this shared philosophy, it makes business sense to be a responsible member of the community.

Community involvement can be achieved through numerous methods. For instance, medical practices can sponsor health fairs to educate the local community regarding important health issues. Charitable care is also another way to interact with the local community. These experiences can also be leveraged through local media outlets; however, care should be taken so that media attention does not overshadow the charitable efforts.

■ Analysis of Community Health Risks

For a medical practice to meet the needs of the health care community, it has to ascertain what those needs are. To do so, a systematic process for describing and quantifying the risks associated with a particular health problem and the possible consequences should be established.[110] A step-by-step procedure can be utilized to conduct an assessment of the health risks present in a particular community. The first step is to define the health care community and identify key individuals and organizations. Particular attention should be given to achieving broad representation and include individuals with diverse viewpoints regarding problems and solutions.[111]

Engaging Partners

Medical practice executives need to develop creative and flexible methods to engage partners and community members in a conversation regarding community health risks. One strategy that may be employed is to schedule meetings at different times and locations, employing a variety of methods including town forums, conference calls, and anonymous surveys.[112]

Collecting Data

An excellent first step in the data collection process is to access community health data via community and state government Websites. Often, these Websites offer a plethora of secondary data, eliminating the need to collect firsthand or primary data. However, sometimes additional quantitative and qualitative data are necessary to present a complete picture of a particular community's health risks.[113]

Developing Health Priorities

Once data have been compiled and analyzed, the medical practice executive should engage community partners and members of the community in a stakeholder conversation to establish criteria so that priority areas can be identified. Once criteria have been established, the list of health risks present in the community can be ranked.[114]

Clarifying the Issue

To gain a clear understanding of the health risks, it is necessary to explore factors that contribute to the problem and determine which aspect of the problem is actually the area of concern. It is often necessary to collect additional data to understand the relationship between a health indicator, the available resources, and other influential factors.

Implementation Plan

Once this groundwork has been set, the medical practice executive should consider strategy and develop an implementation plan. Rather than reinventing the wheel, successful strategies utilized in other communities should be considered. The key to implementation is selecting a course of action that is manageable and evaluating the course of action to ensure success.

■ Wellness/Health Benchmarks

To judge the success of community health interventions, the medical practice executive should compare local results with national or state campaigns. One such national resource is *Healthy People 2010*, which is a comprehensive set of disease prevention and health promotion objectives for the nation to achieve by 2010.[115] In addition, most states have established health benchmarks for communities to achieve.

To assess the effectiveness of addressing community health risks, the medical practice executive can conduct periodic surveys and compare them to state and national-level efforts. By comparing the results of local health care efforts with state and national surveys, behavioral change can be assessed. When gaps in progress are identified, efforts can be redirected to help achieve better disease management results.

■ Public Relations Methods

Just like other forms of marketing, public relations should also have a carefully structured plan. Effective methods for promoting a medical practice's name and services include conducting an open house, participating in speakers bureaus, authoring newspaper articles and columns, posting Website presentations, and creating physician referral newsletters.

Open Houses

Open houses provide an excellent reason to invite customers and referral sources to your medical group practice. Open houses can be used to introduce new physicians, highlight new services, or celebrate a milestone within the medical practice. Members of the media from the local newspaper as well as radio and television stations should be included so that good relationships can be established. Establishing positive relationships with media outlets is essential in being able to leverage and influence present and future media coverage.[116]

Speakers Bureaus

Participating in speakers bureaus can be an effective part of a medical practice's public relations efforts. Speakers bureaus present the opportunity to communicate the practice's marketing message to a captive audience. Often, speaking engagements are publicized and covered by the media, increasing their value as a public relations tool.[117]

Newspaper Columns

The printed word is an effective method to support public relations activities. Newspapers provide a cost-free forum for medical practice executives and physicians to share their opinions and expertise to the community-at-large.

Website Presentations

Using the Internet for advertising and promoting a medical practice has become commonplace. Developing a Website helps the practices to describe its offerings and also delivers the message that the organization is up-to-date and on the cutting edge. Done properly, Website presentation can be an effective tool for exposure.

Physician Referral Newsletters

Fact sheets, physician referral newsletters, and brochures can be tailored to support public relations. Printed material provides the necessary facts about the medical practice and its services to prospective clients as well as to other physicians who may be unaware of the practice's offerings. Brochures can be created and printed in-house so that costs can be reduced and the content can be changed easily as necessary.

Publicity

Publicity refers to free communication of information about an organization's facility and available services, which is an integral part of the organization's public relations strategy. Because publicity is free, this method for reaching the community and customers should be leveraged.

Opportunities for publicity can be categorized into three general areas:

1. News releases;

2. Media coverage; and

3. Medical media opportunities.

News Releases

The media plays an important informational role in community outreach opportunities. Members of the local media are continually searching for public health information activities as part of their public service mission.[118]

Medical group practices can develop news releases by partnering with the local media to highlight events occurring at the facility, or perhaps to highlight outstanding staff members. For example, a practice may want to develop a news release showcasing new technology that the practice offers, or perhaps a physician who received a national recognition award.

Media Coverage

An excellent method to ensure media coverage is to identify human interest stories. Medical practice executives need to be creative and identify events that are of interest to the community. One such event may be how staff members are participating in charity work, such as physicians volunteering at local charities providing health care to the homeless and uninsured. Another example may include media coverage of a health fair sponsored by the medical practice. Further means to generate media coverage can be accomplished by organizing programs and special events to which the public is invited.[119]

Medical Media Opportunities

It is important for the medical practice executive to leverage media opportunities to help market the practice's services. Some opportunities include working with local radio and television stations to provide medical information, or celebrating and taking advantage of nationally recognized efforts, such as Patient Safety Awareness Week or the American Heart Month, by creating and/or sponsoring public service announcements with local media outlets. Another cost-free method is encouraging clinical staff members to write editorials and op-ed pieces for local papers and newsletters.[120]

■ Internal Relations

It is important to maintain effective communications and relations with external customers, but it is also crucial to communicate with internal customers. Practice executives cannot overlook the importance of their employees and physician owners. In other words, if the medical practice executive takes care of the employees, the employees will take care of the patients. Several methods ensure effective communications with employees, including writing a staff newsletter, regular staff meetings, establishing an intranet, and suggestion boxes.

Staff Newsletter

A staff newsletter can be a vehicle for regular communication with the staff and key stakeholders. Newsletters are an excellent method to reinforce organizational goals and objectives. By using targeted articles, practice executives can include employee success stories that highlight steps in the right direction. The story not only acts as reinforcement, but it also provides employees with recognition.

Another purpose a staff newsletter serves is to provide employees with a periodic update on the current state of affairs. For instance, if part of the practice's goals is to provide on-time service, each newsletter could show the trend toward that goal, along with ideas to help continue a positive trend or new ideas to turn around a negative trend. Another excellent idea is to provide a year-end report to show the practice's final results for each objective. The newsletter can be another method to communicate important information to staff, rather than the traditional meeting or memo.

Staff Meetings

Staff meetings can be an effective way to maintain communication within an organization. These meetings should be viewed as learning opportunities for practice executives and their staff. Meetings can increase the effectiveness and bottom line of both large and small practices, but if not properly conducted, however, meetings can waste staff time.

Meetings should therefore have a purpose and a defined agenda. The practice executive should keep the meeting on-task; otherwise, participants will lose focus and dread future meetings. Another method to increase the productivity of meetings is to provide staff members with the agenda in advance of the meeting, so they can research the topics for discussion. When staff members are properly prepared, meetings can be effective vehicles for problem solving. One last tip is to follow up all meetings with a thoughtful note to attendees to summarize meeting accomplishments and action plans. This note is more personal than simple meeting minutes sent by e-mail, which typically are deleted without ever being read.

Intranet Communication

An intranet is an internal network belonging to an organization and is typically accessible only by the organization's members. Like the Internet, intranets provide access to information; however, they are secure from unauthorized users and provide organizations with their own personal information resource. Intranet sites can be used to inform stakeholders of what is happening in the practice, changes in practice procedures, upcoming training sessions, continuing education unit (CEU) opportunities, and updates on new governmental regulations. They can also provide links for help.

Suggestion Boxes

Suggestion boxes no longer have to be of the wooden variety. Currently, electronic suggestion boxes are often located on an organization's Website and also may be found on its intranet. The suggestion box located on the external Website, which is accessible via the Internet, can serve to solicit opinions, experiences, and perceptions of customers. Perhaps more important is the suggestion box located within the organization's intranet. Frequently, employees have the knowledge and information necessary to improve the organization; however, they withhold the information for fear of reprisal. This method of communication, if anonymous, can overcome that objection.

■ Stakeholder Identification and Management

Stakeholders include any individuals or organizations that have an interest in the success of the organization. They can be classified as internal, external, or interface stakeholders. The term "internal stakeholder" refers to any individual who works wholly within the organization, such as office staff. External stakeholders refer to individuals and organizations that function outside of the organization, such as vendors, patients, and other physician practices. Interface stakeholders are those who function both internally and externally, such as hospital medical staff. Interface stakeholders tend to be quite rare when discussing most types of medical group practices.[121]

Needs/Expectations

The needs and desires of these stakeholders influence the strategy of an organization. Not all stakeholders are equal in terms of their power and influence; in fact some wield incredible power, whereas others are virtually powerless. Thus, it is necessary to understand the specific demands of each stakeholder so that they can be addressed and satisfied.

Customized Communications

Just like the previously mentioned methods of communicating with internal stakeholders, it is necessary to develop direct communications for external and interface stakeholders. Methods of communicating with this audience include targeted e-mails, direct mailings and newsletters, and conference calls.

■ Survey Techniques

An effective method of determining customers' needs can be accomplished through the use of survey research. Surveys can also be effective tools to test new ideas or gauge interest in new services as well as to help evaluate a practice's operation. The most common types of surveys are conducted via mail, telephone, or face-to-face – each method having its own advantages and disadvantages.[122]

Mail and E-mail Surveys

Mail surveys are conducted, as the name suggests, via the U.S. Postal Service. Typically, the organization sends surveys to a target audience, and the respondents return them using prepaid, self-addressed envelopes supplied with the surveys. Less expensive surveys can be conducted via e-mail. Inexpensive online resources are available that can assist in the development, collection, and the analysis of results.[123]

The primary advantage of mail and e-mail surveys is the ability to target a large number of respondents with little effort. The major disadvantage is that response rates to mail and e-mail surveys can be quite low. Another potential disadvantage is that respondents may not understand the intent of survey questions and thus may respond inappropriately. This problem is inherent in all surveys and can be minimized by thoroughly pilot-testing the survey to help ensure comprehension.[124]

Telephone Surveys

For a telephone survey, a target audience is selected and contacted by telephone until enough responses have been obtained. The primary advantages of telephone surveys are that they are low in cost and offer the advantage of being able to personally clarify the intention of survey questions. Another advantage is that response rates are typically higher than those received for surface mail or e-mail surveys. Major disadvantages are that telephone surveys are time-intensive and that contact with those on the list is not guaranteed because respondents may not be at home or answer the telephone. Despite the fact that telephone survey response is higher than that for mail surveys, there is usually a high degree of refusal to cooperate.[125]

In-Person Surveys

In-person surveys are conducted face-to-face. An effective method for delivering surveys is to provide patients with surveys during the registration process. A well-designed survey can help patients pass the time until they are called and can help collect valuable information. An advantage of face-to-face surveys, as with telephone surveys, is that the intent of the questions can be clarified. A downside to face-to-face surveys is the perceived lack of anonymity. One solution to this is to have a locked response box for the return of surveys.

■ Culture of Customer Service

A necessary part of interacting with internal and external customers is to project a positive image. One method to achieve this is to instill in your organization a culture of customer service, meaning that all employees should strive to meet and exceed customers' needs, both internally and externally. To do this, medical practice executives need to take the lead and outline expectations; otherwise, the concept of customer service is left open for individual interpretation.

If expectations for delivering customer service and a culture of customer service are not outlined, when a problem surfaces, there is a risk of not only losing a customer, but the practice executive is also faced with reprimanding an employee.[126] These potential issues can be avoided through clear policies and procedures or through initial and ongoing training seminars.

Organizational cultures exist either consciously or subconsciously. Practice executives have the power to choose and shape the culture they want to work within and to transmit that vision to employees and customers. Unfortunately, the culture of customer service doesn't happen overnight, or even in a month. Training can support the change process, but a culture shift requires that internal customers (employees) treat one another with the same dignity and respect that they would award to a guest, and that they trust each other to do the job.[127]

To instill a culture of customer service, practice executives must provide employees with training and the basic tools to deliver customer service. Some topic suggestions include telephone etiquette, reception desk protocol, cellular phone etiquette, dealing with difficult and demanding patients, and effective bedside manner.

Telephone Etiquette

Telephones are an essential tool for communication; however, few individuals are versed in their proper use. When answering a business phone, employees should always clearly identify the name of the organization as well as themselves. All too often, employees either forget to do so, or speak so quickly that the name of the organization is unrecognizable. The medical practice executive should develop standard protocols that outline the manner in which phones are answered. Often it is necessary to place callers on hold to deal with patients in person. The protocols should include always asking permission before putting the caller on hold and, after returning to them, thanking them for waiting, and completing the conversation. Conversely, when an employee is talking to a patient face-to-face, that conversation should never be interrupted to take a telephone call – that is the purpose of answering machines.[128]

The medical practice executive should emphasize to the staff that when making outgoing phone calls, the key is to respect the caller's time. For example, when making calls to confirm appointments or convey information, staff should always ask whether it is a convenient time to interrupt. Then the caller should deliver the message, answer any questions, and end the conversation.

Cellular Phone Etiquette

Cellular phones are convenient; however, they can invariably interrupt at the most inopportune moments. Policies need to be developed to govern their use in the practice.

Reception Desk Etiquette

"You never get a second chance to make a first impression" is obviously true when a patient encounters the receptionists. Receptionists should always exhibit proper manners. When a person enters the practice, the receptionist should immediately welcome the visitor using a normal tone of voice. All too often, receptionists are either too busy to say "hello," or they tend to "bark out" orders. When possible, receptionists should attempt to use surnames to convey a message of respect to customers. When notifying patients that the "doctor is ready," all efforts should be made to do so in a friendly and calm manner, keeping in mind the patient's ability to react quickly.

Dealing with Difficult People

Often, health care personnel are confronted with difficult people. A primary reason for this is that most patients would rather be somewhere else, and they are anxious about the outcome of their treatment. When encountering individuals who are difficult or defensive, the staff needs to recognize that it is futile to confront such people. They should keep in mind that these persons are insecure and their demeanor is not personal. The staff members should maintain their composure, allow the person to vent, and attempt to provide assistance. One strategy to deal with a difficult person is to empathize with the person and empower him or her by presenting available options to help resolve the matter. If the person becomes abusive, the staff member may consider asking someone else to intercede to deal with the person, or even inviting the person to leave.

Effective Bedside Manner

To deliver customer service excellence, every person in the medical practice must present a caring and genuine manner. This is especially important in the physician-patient relationship. Although physicians are trained to pay attention to patients' emotions and concerns, the realities and time pressures of medical practice make this task difficult. Physicians do not have time to listen to a litany of the patient's psychological complaints, so the strategy often is to "get in there, get the facts, and get out" as soon as possible.[129] Effective bedside manner, however, requires that physicians consider their patients' emotional, social, and family situations. Delivering patient care with a personal touch has tremendous rewards – when patients feel secure and supported, their health is more likely to improve.[130] Physicians need to remember the reasons why they chose health care as a career and to project an attitude of care during every patient encounter.

■ Conclusion

Developing community outreach, public relations, and customer relations programs is an essential part of any marketing strategy. It is not necessary for medical practices to engage in all of the strategies presented here to be successful. What *is* necessary, however, is that the practice executive communicates a well-defined strategy to the staff in order to meet the demands of the community being served.

Conclusion

SUCCESSFUL MEDICAL PRACTICE EXECUTIVES will be those who embrace strategic planning and marketing, rather than those who are merely reactive to their environments. Strategic planning allows the practice to change direction in a quick and consistent fashion and can help medical group practices achieve goals and objectives on a continuous basis, especially as they relate to a rapidly changing, dynamic environment. Adaptability is key for medical practice executives to survive and thrive in the turbulent and complex change of pace in health care.

Additionally, the growth of consumerism and the technological changes to the delivery of health care pose challenges to medical groups. Medical practice executives are (and will be) continually exposed to an arsenal of marketing tools to take advantage of these opportunities. An effective marketing plan incorporates much of the information of the strategic and business plans, but shifts the focus to the external environment.

It is not enough to simply develop strategic, business, and marketing plans; rather, medical practice executives must continually monitor and evaluate the planning activities and the status of plan implementation. This volume showed practice executives a systematic method for measuring the effectiveness of these plans, which must be established so that clear links between past, present, and future strategies and results can be determined.

Additionally, monitoring and evaluation can help medical practice executives to extract relevant information from past and ongoing activities that can subsequently be used for fine-tuning strategies. Without a formal process for monitoring and evaluation, it would be impossible to assess the effectiveness of current strategies and how to improve future efforts.

Furthermore, to prosper in today's health care market, a group practice must employ a long-term strategy that is driven by commitment, continuity, and consistency so that its relationship with the community can be sustained. Medical practice managers must build trust and commitment within the community and among the customers they serve. To do so, medical practices need to become actively engaged in the community in which they operate.

Medical practice executives must have a vision of the past, present, and future; they must succeed in communicating such a vision to others in a way that the followers adopt their vision as their own.

Exercises

THESE QUESTIONS have been retired from the ACMPE Essay Exam question bank. Because there are so many ways to handle various situations, there are no "right" answers and, thus, no answer key. Use these questions to help you practice responses in different scenarios.

1. You are the administrator of a four-physician orthopedic practice in a rural area. The physicians travel to 15 satellite clinics in order to meet the needs of referring physicians and patients. Several physicians believe that they are not seeing a sufficient number of patients to justify their travel time and are considering the elimination of some sites.

    Discuss how you would help the physicians arrive at a decision.

2. You are the administrator of a medical practice. One of the physicians in your group is interested in setting up an outreach clinic at a hospital in a neighboring community.

    Explain how you would evaluate this proposal.

3. You are the administrator of a medical practice. Your practice has been functioning primarily on a "cross that bridge when we get to it" basis. In light of increasing competition and declining patient base, you believe a formal strategic planning retreat is critical. Many of the physicians in the practice have grown accustomed to the current system and may oppose this planning session.

   Describe how you would engage the physicians in the strategic planning process.

4. You are the administrator of a five-physician medical prac-
    tice. Your board of directors has decided to double the
    number of providers within the practice. At its next meet-
    ing, the board would like you to propose a plan of action to
    accomplish this goal.

    Describe how you would develop this plan of action and
    discuss the plan's critical components.

5. You are the administrator of a medical group practice and
    are in charge of coordinating the group's annual planning
    retreat. Physicians in your group have complained that pre-
    vious retreats amounted to nothing more than another
    board meeting. It is your responsibility to ensure a produc-
    tive and focused retreat that will result in identifying the
    group's strategic initiatives consistent with its vision and
    mission.

    Describe your plan of action for the retreat.

6. You are the administrator of a medical practice. The group is comprised of equal numbers of physicians at various stages of their careers. The group is facing several strategic issues/challenges. When the executive committee meets, it becomes involved in endless discussions with only peripheral relevance to the issues. Few decisions are produced, and the more senior physician leaders dominate the discussion with little input from the junior members.

Describe how you would handle this situation.

7. You are the administrator of a six-physician, single-specialty medical practice. The practice grew over a period of 20 years, and until two years ago, it was the only practice for this specialty in the immediate and surrounding area. Your service area comprises several small to mid-sized communities. About two years ago, competition to your practice emerged in one of the nearby communities. Additionally, you have become increasingly concerned about the decline in gross revenue resulting from patients transferring out of the practice and the lack of new patient registrations and referrals.

   Describe how you would handle this situation.

8. You are the administrator of a busy 12-provider orthopedic practice. Your medical group is well established within your community, and over the past several years it has experienced strong referral patterns from most of the community's primary care practices. One of your senior surgeons has come to you with concerns that he has noticed a decrease in referrals from two primary care practices. He tells you he thinks several of the former primary care physicians retired, and he has noticed that the new physicians do not seem to be referring as many patients to him. He has asked you for specific recommendations to address the problem.

    Describe how you would handle this situation.

9. You are the administrator of a 35-physician multispecialty group in a metropolitan area. During the past year, patient visits have decreased by 20 percent. Several members of the executive committee believe that there has been a shift in market share to other new physicians who have moved to the community. Other board members believe that the shift has been a result of poor patient service. The board has asked you to develop a specific plan of action to reverse this trend.

Describe how you would handle this situation.

10. You are the administrator of a satellite facility for a multi-specialty group practice, which is located in a suburb approximately 25 miles from the central facility. The satellite is staffed with eight family practitioners, two nurse practitioners, and rotating specialists from the main facility. The satellite practice serves a different payer mix than the overall medical group. A small multispecialty practice from a neighboring suburb recently opened a new facility within a mile of your site. While your payer contracts are secure, several of the payers have been offering point-of-service products with open provider panels. These products have experienced significant growth. You are concerned that you will lose market share to the competing multispecialty group and have discussed the situation with the physicians at your site.

Describe how you would further address this situation.

11. You are the chief operating officer of a 17-physician single-specialty practice. Three years ago, your market was heavily penetrated by health maintenance organizations (HMOs), paying physicians on a capitation basis. At that time, your physician group sold its 15-year-old practice to a Physician Practice Management Company (PPMC). The PPMC employs all of your group's physicians, the staff, and yourself. The practice was moved to a facility owned and financed by the PPMC. The PPMC just notified the physicians that the corporation is divesting its ownership of physician practices. The company has given you 120 days' notice of its intent to sell the practice. The physicians have requested that you investigate buying the practice back. You have 45 days to complete this work.

Describe how you would handle this situation.

12. You are the administrator employed by a primary care medical practice that is owned by a nonprofit community hospital. The medical practice is losing more than $50,000 per full-time equivalent (FTE) physician per year. Discussions are taking place with the hospital concerning severing the relationship. Your physicians respect your vision and leadership, and have asked for your opinion regarding the future direction of the group. They have asked you to evaluate the group's options and make a recommendation at the next board meeting.

Describe how you would handle this situation.

Notes

1. B. C. Johnson & J. J. Erlsland, "Development of a Strategic Planning Process for Multi-Department Management in a Medical Center," *Journal of the American Dietetic Association* 99, no. 9, Supplement 1 (1983).

2. Douglas A. Singh, *Effective Management of Long-Term Care Facilities* (Sudbury, Mass.: Jones and Bartlett Publishers, 2005).

3. Sharon B. Buchbinder, Modena Wilson, Clifford F. Melick, Neil R. Powe. "Primary Care Physician Job Satisfaction and Turnover." *American Journal of Managed Care* (July 2001): 701–713.

4. The U.S. Census Bureau, "Income, Poverty, and Health Insurance Coverage in the United States: 2003," www.census.gov/hhes/ www/hlthin03.html.

5. Christina Pope, "Connect with Your Community: How Outreach Can Strengthen Your Practice," *MGMA Connexion* 4, no. 10 (2004): 30–35.

6. Robert J. Stevens, "Going to Market," *Marketing Health Services* (Summer 2005): 26–31.

7. Johnson & Erlsland, "Development of a Strategic Planning Process for Multi-Department Management in a Medical Center."

8. Robert C. Shirley, "Strategic Planning: An Overview," *Successful Strategic Planning: Case Studies, New Directions for Higher Education* 64 (Winter 1982): 5–14.

9. J. Max Reiboldt, "Writing a Group Practice Business Plan," *Healthcare Financial Management* (July 1999): 58–61.

10. Timothy Rotarius & Dawn Oetjen, "Dialysis Center Alliances," *Dialysis & Transplantation* 31, no. 3 (2002): 151–154.

11. Richard A. D'Aveni, *Hypercompetition: Managing the Dynamics of Strategic Maneuvering* (New York: Free Press, 1994).

12. Clarkson Centre for Business Ethics, *Principles of Stakeholder Management* (Toronto, Ont.: Clarkson Centre for Business Ethics, 1999).

13. Arnold D. Kaluzny & Howard S. Zuckerman, "Alliances in a Changing Industry," in *The 21st Century Health Care Leader*, Roderick W. Gilkey, ed. (San Francisco: Jossey-Bass, 1999), 149–157.

14. Singh, *Effective Management of Long-Term Care Facilities*.

15. Henry Mintzberg, *The Rise and Fall of Strategic Planning* (New York: The Free Press, 1994), 12.

16. Russell L. Ackoff, *A Concept of Corporate Planning* (New York: Wiley-Interscience, 1970); Mintzberg, *The Rise and Fall of Strategic Planning*, 11.

17. Arnoldo C. Hax & Nicolas S. Majluf, *The Strategy Concept and Process: A Pragmatic Approach* (Upper Saddle River, N.J.: Prentice Hall, 1996), 14.

18. John M. Bryson, *Strategic Planning for Public and Nonprofit Organizations: A Guide to Strengthening and Sustaining Organizational Achievement* (San Francisco: Jossey-Bass, 2004).

19. T. J. Rowley, "Moving beyond Didactic Ties: A Network of Stakeholder Influences," *Academy of Management Review* 22, no. 4 (1997): 887–910.

20. Linda E. Swayne, Peter M. Ginter, & W. Jack Duncan, *The Physician Strategist: Setting a Strategic Direction for Your Practice* (Chicago: Irwin Professional Publishing, 1996).

21. Carter McNamara, *Field Guide to Nonprofit Strategic Planning and Facilitation* (Minneapolis, Minn.: Authenticity Consulting, LLC, 2000).

22. Ibid.

23. Edgar H. Schein, *Organizational Culture and Leadership* (San Francisco: Jossey-Bass, 1988).

24. Bryson, *Strategic Planning for Public and Nonprofit Organizations*.

25. Medical Group Management Association, "Mission, Vision and Values," www.mgma.com (retrieved August 18, 2005); Merck & Co., Inc, "Mission Statement," www.merck.com/about/mission.html (retrieved August 18, 2005).

26. Bryson, *Strategic Planning for Public and Nonprofit Organizations*.

27. McNamara, *Field Guide to Nonprofit Strategic Planning and Facilitation*.

28. Ibid.

29. Susan R. Lambreth, *Don't Just Plan – Implement: Steps to Successful Practice Group Plans*, Hildebrandt International Publications. https://www.hildebrandt.com/Documents.aspx?Doc_ID=1938 (retrieved August 18, 2005).

30. Ibid.

31. JIAN Tools for Sales, "Components of a Business Plan," www.jian.com/software/business-plan/write-a-business-plan/Components.htm (retrieved August 18, 2005).

32. "Elements of a Business Plan," *Entrepreneur.com Magazine*, 2001, www.entrepreneur.com/article/0,4621,287355,00.html (retrieved August 18, 2005).

33. Ibid.

34. Ibid.

35. Ibid.

36. JIAN Tools for Sales, "Components of a Business Plan."

37. PlanWare, "White Paper: Writing a Business Plan," www.planware.org/bizplan.htm (retrieved August 18, 2005).

38. Louis E. Boone & David L. Kurtz, *Contemporary Marketing Wired*, 3rd Edition (New York: Dryden Press, 1998).

39. Michael E. Porter, *Competitive Strategy* (New York: The Free Press, New York, 1980).

40. American Marketing Association, "Marketing Definitions," www.marketingpower.com/ (1995; retrieved September 9, 2005).

41. Meir Liraz, "Managing a Small Business," www.liraz.com/marketing.htm (1998; retrieved September 10, 2005).

42. Ibid.

43. "Market Strategies," *Entrepreneur.com Magazine*, www.entrepreneur.com/article/0,4621,270370,00.html (2004; retrieved August 18, 2005).

44. Ibid.

45. Gather the People, "Training Guide #7: Organizational Structure and Culture," www.gatherthepeople.org/Downloads/007_STRUCTURE_CULTURE.pdf (2004; retrieved September 13, 2005).

46. Ibid.

47. Azad N. Hosein, *A Framework for Monitoring and Evaluation in a Public or Private-Sector Environment* (Project Management Institute, Southern Caribbean Chapter, Trinidad, W.I.: 2003).

48. Ibid.

49. Willie Lujan & Edmund Gomez, "Monitoring and Evaluating a Business' Value-Added Effort," http://ag.arizona.edu/arec/va/mon&eval.html (2000; retrieved September 2, 2005).

50. McNamara, *Field Guide to Nonprofit Strategic Planning and Facilitation*.

51. Hosein, *A Framework for Monitoring and Evaluation in a Public or Private-Sector Environment.*

52. Lujan and Gomez, "Monitoring and Evaluating a Business' Value-Added Effort."

53. Ibid.

54. Inter-American Development Bank, "Evaluation – A Management Tool for Improving Project Performance," www.iadb.org/cont/evo (1997; retrieved August 18, 2005).

55. McNamara, *Field Guide to Nonprofit Strategic Planning and Facilitation.*

56. Hosein, *A Framework for Monitoring and Evaluation in a Public or Private-Sector Environment.*

57. S. Anderson, "In Today's Economy (and Tomorrow's), Strategic Alliances Open Doors to Opportunities," *Orange County Business Journal* 25, no. 4 (January 28-February 3, 2002): 4.

58. John R. Harbison and Peter Pekar, *A Practical Guide to Repeatable Success* (San Francisco: Jossey-Bass, 1998).

59. Rotarius and Oetjen, "Dialysis Center Alliances."

60. Ibid.

61. Peter R. Kongstvedt, David W. Plocher, & Jean C. Stanford, "Integrated Health Care Delivery Systems," in *Essentials of Managed Health Care*, 4th Edition, Peter R. Kongstvedt, ed. (Gaithersburg, Md.: Aspen Publishers, Inc., 2001), 31–62.

62. Michael K. Rich, "Requirements for Successful Marketing Alliances," *The Journal of Business and Industrial Marketing* 18, no. 4/5 (2003): 447–457.

63. Thomas M. Finn & David A McCamey, "P&G's Guide to Successful Partnerships," *Pharmaceutical Executive* 22, no. 1 (January 2002): 54–60.

64. Rich, "Requirements for Successful Marketing Alliances."

65. Salvatore Parise & Lisa Sasson, "Leveraging Knowledge Management across Strategic Alliances," *Ivey Business Journal* 66, no. 4 (March/April 2002): 41–47.

66. Kongstvedt, Plocher, and Stanford, "Integrated Health Care Delivery Systems."

67. Peter M. Ginter, Linda E. Swayne, & W. Jack Duncan, *Strategic Management of Health Care Organizations*, 4th Edition (Malden, Mass.: Blackwell Publishing Inc., 2002), 240.

68. Alan M. Zuckerman, "Strategic Alliances and Joint Ventures: Why Make When You Can Buy?" *Healthcare Financial Management* 59, no. 8 (2005): 122–124.

69. Ibid.

70. Kongstvedt, Plocher, and Stanford, "Integrated Health Care Delivery Systems."

71. Ibid.

72. Ibid.

73. Ibid.

74. Ibid.

75. Ibid.

76. Ibid.

77. Ibid.

78. Ibid.

79. Ibid.

80. Ibid.

81. Ibid.

82. Ibid.

83. Ibid.

84. Rod Aymond & Theodore Hariton, "Regrouping after Disintegration," *Family Practice Management* 7, no. 3 (2000): 37–40.

85. Kriss Barlow & Allison McCarthy, "Due Diligence on the Internal Front Enhances Recruiting Success," *The New England Journal of Medicine* (January-February 2004).

86. Ibid.

87. United States Agency for International Development (USAID), "Due Diligence for Private Enterprise," www.usaid.gov/our_work/global_partnerships (retrieved October 17, 2005).

88. Ibid.

89. Ibid.

90. Aymond and Hariton, "Regrouping after Disintegration."

91. Ibid.

92. Ibid.

93. Parise and Sasson, "Leveraging Knowledge Management across Strategic Alliances."

94. Rich, "Requirements for Successful Marketing Alliances."

95. James G. March & Zur Shapira, "Managerial Perspectives on Risk and Risk Taking" *Management Science* 33 (1987): 1404–1418.

96. John Hagedoorn, "Understanding the Rationale of Strategic Technology Partnering: Interorganizational Modes of Cooperation and Sectoral Differences," *Strategic Management Journal* 14 (1993): 371–385; B. Kogut, "Joint Ventures: Theoretical and Empirical Perspectives, *Strategic Management Journal* 9 (1988): 319–332.

97. Oliver E. Williamson, "Credible Commitments: Using Hostages to Support Exchange," *American Economic Review* 73 (1983): 519–540; Oliver E. Williamson, *The Economic Institutions of Capitalism* (New York: Free Press, 1985).

98. Anderson, "In Today's Economy (and Tomorrow's), Strategic Alliances Open Doors to Opportunities."

99. Ibid.

100. Clarkson Centre for Ethics & Board Effectiveness, "Redefining the Corporation: Publications: Principles of Stakeholder Management," www.Mgmt.utoronto.ca/~stake.Publications.htm.

101. Ibid.

102. Ibid.

103. Ibid.

104. Ibid.

105. Stephanie J. Lee, Anthony L. Back, Susan D. Block, & Susan K. Stewart, "Enhancing Physician-Patient Communication," *Hematology: American Society of Hematology Education Program*: 464–483, www.entrepreneur.com/article/0,4621,310647,00.html (retrieved September 17, 2005).

106. Office for the Advancement of Telehealth, "Welcome Page," telehealth.hrsa.gov/welcome.htm (retrieved October 18, 2005).

107. Ibid.

108. M. Tervalon & J. Murray-Garcia, "Cultural Humility vs. Cultural Competence: A Critical Distinction in Defining Physician Training Outcomes in Medical Education," *Journal of Health Care Poor Underserved* 9 (1998):117–125.

109. Ibid.

110. Vincent T. Covello & Miley W. Merkhofer, *Risk Assessment Methods: Approaches for Assessing Health and Environmental Risks* (New York: Plenum Press, 1993).

111. New York State Department of Health (NYSDOH), New York State Community Health Assessment (CHA) Guidance Documents, www. health.state.ny.us/nysdoh/chac (retrieved October 19, 2005).

112. Ibid.

113. Ibid.

114. Ibid.

115. U.S. Department of Health and Human Services. *Healthy People 2010*, 2nd Edition. With *Understanding and Improving Health,* and *Objectives for Improving Health.* 2 Vols. Washington, D.C.: U.S. Government Printing Office, November 2000.

116. Al Lautenslager, "PR Is More Than Just Press Releases," www.entrepreneur. com/article/0,4621,310647,00.html (2003; retrieved October 19, 2005).

117. Ibid.

118. National Association of City and County Health Officials (NACCHO), "NACCHO Public Health Communications Toolkit," http://archive.naccho. org/documents/Communication-toolkit.pdf (retrieved September 18, 2005).

119. Ibid.

120. Ibid.

121. Myron D. Fottler, John D. Blair, J. D. Whitehead, M. D. Luas, & G. T. Savage, "Assessing Key Stakeholders: Who Matters to Hospitals and Why?" *Hospital and Health Services Administration* 34, no. 4 (1989): 527.

122. Ryerson University, "Survey Techniques," www.ryerson.ca/~mjoppe/ ResearchProcess (retrieved September 20, 2005).

123. American Statistical Society (ASA), "ASA Series: What Is a Survey?" www.amstat.org/sections/srms/brochures (retrieved September 20, 2005).

124. Ibid.

125. Ryerson University, "Survey Techniques."

126. Carol Verret, "Creating a Culture of Customer Service," www.hotel-online. com/Trends/CarolVerret (2000; retrieved September 20, 2005).

127. Ibid.

128. California State University, Fullerton, "Telephone Etiquette," www. fullerton.edu/it/services (retrieved September 18, 2005).

129. Kim Mulvihill, "Bedside Manner," www.sfgate.com/cgi-bin/article. cgi?file= (2001; retrieved September 11, 2005).

130. Ibid.

Glossary

Alliances – A form of cooperative arrangement between two or more physician groups or between physicians and hospitals.

Assets – Everything a company or person owns or is owed, such as money, securities, equipment, and buildings. Assets are listed on a company's balance sheet.

Balance sheet – A summary of financial information broken down into three areas: (1) assets, (2) liabilities, and (3) equity.

Balanced Scorecard system – A strategic management approach that translates a vision into a clear set of objectives or critical success factors.

Bank-financing plan – A plan that focuses on persuading the banker that the practice can satisfy its needs through historical financial ratios, assets, and so forth.

Baseline indicators – Established measures used to determine how well an organization is meeting its customers' needs as well as other operational and financial performance expectations.

Benchmark – A standard by which something can be measured or judged.

Business plan – A document that defines the practice, identifies its goals, and serves as its operational resume.

Cash flow statement – A statement that demonstrates how much cash will be needed to meet obligations, when the cash is going to be required, and its source.

Communication competency – The demonstration of communication skills necessary to elicit multiple points of view from internal and external sources, to facilitate constructive interaction, and to present information clearly and concisely.

Competitive advantage – The means by which the practice seeks to differentiate itself from other similar practices.

Competitive pricing – A pricing strategy used by practices that are entering a market where there is already an established price and it is difficult to differentiate one product from another.

Consumer analysis – An analysis that explores the demographic makeup of the practice's consumer base, but also delves a bit deeper into the consumers' purchasing and decision-making behaviors, their motivation and expectations, and loyalty segments.

Conventional planning – Planning oriented toward looking at problems based on current understanding, or an inside-out mind-set.

Cost-plus pricing – A pricing plan that assures that all costs, both fixed and variable, are covered and the desired profit percentage is attained.

Current assets – Assets that will be converted to cash or will be used by the practice in a year or less.

Current liabilities – Liabilities that are due in one year or less.

Demand pricing – A pricing plan used by practices that sell their services and/or products through a variety of sources at differing prices, based on demand.

Due diligence – A process that entails collecting information and data in order to assess the feasibility of a particular venture so that a decision is reached only after considering all prudent viewpoints.

Equity – The difference between total assets and total liabilities.

Executive summary – A nontechnical summary statement designed to provide a quick overview of the full-length report on which it is based.

External stakeholder – A group related, but external, to a practice that includes suppliers, investors, community groups, and government organizations.

Evaluation – A process that attempts to determine, as systematically and objectively as possible, the relevance, effectiveness, efficiency, and impact (both intentional and unintentional) of plans in the context of their stated objectives.

Financial business plan – A plan that allows potential lending sources to view the practice's ongoing financial status, risk, past and future spending habits, and prospects before committing funds.

Fixed assets – Assets that will last for more than one year.

4Ps – Product (what the actual offering comprises), price (the value exchanged for that offering), promotion (the means of communicating that offering to the target audience, promotional mix), and place (also known as distribution, the means of having the product offering available to the target audience). Also known as the marketing mix.

Goals – Specific, measurable, attainable, realistic, time-bound statements that provide the overall context for what the organization is trying to accomplish.

Group Practice Without Walls (GPWW) – A legal merging of all assets of the physician practice.

Impact indicator – Specific information or evidence that can be gathered to measure progress toward program goals and objectives or to measure the effectiveness of program activities when direct measurement is difficult or impossible.

Income statement – A report on a business's proposed or current cash-generating ability.

Independent provider association (IPA) – Association formed to organize independent medical group practices into contracting entities for the purpose of contracting with health maintenance organizations (HMOs) and the purchasing of supplies or other services.

Internal stakeholder – A group directly related to a practice that includes management, staff, administrators, etc.

Joint venture – The combination of the resources of two or more separate organizations to accomplish a designated task.

Leadership competency – A competency of medical practice executives. Leadership is demonstrated by collaborating with and supporting the practice's physician leadership to provide strategic direction to the organization and the operational systems to carry it out.

Liabilities – Anything that is owed to someone else.

Long-term assets – Assets that will last for longer than one year.

Long-term liabilities – Debts that are due in more than one year.

Long-term planning – Planning that represents a projection from the present or an extrapolation from the past.

Macroenvironmental analysis – Continuous structured data collection and processing on a broad range of environmental factors, such as the economy, the governmental and legal environments, technology, and social culture.

Management services organization (MSO) – An organization typically formed to provide management services and administrative systems to one or more medical practices.

Mark-up pricing – Pricing strategy calculated by adding the desired profit to the cost of the product; mainly used by retailers.

Market analysis – Research used to assist in predicting the direction of the markets based on technical data relating to price movements of the market, or on fundamental data such as corporate earnings.

Market position – A practice's relative standing in relation to its competitors.

Marketing – The process of planning and executing the conception, pricing, promotion, and distribution of ideas, goods, services, organizations, and events to create and maintain relationships that will satisfy individual and organizational objectives.

Marketing activities – All activities associated with identifying the particular wants and needs of a target market of customers, and then going about satisfying those customers better than the competition.

Marketing mix – The combination of product offerings used to reach a target market for the organization (also known as the 4Ps).

Marketing plan – A plan that focuses on the external environment and the identification of segments, along with the target market selection, positioning, and development of the 4Ps expected from marketers.

Marketing research – Surveys of the area in which a product or service is to be offered to determine the cost of doing business, any competition, potential sales, and so forth.

Market segmentation – The method of grouping a market into smaller subgroups; the process of target marketing.

Microenvironmental analysis – An analysis that seeks to uncover the resources of the practice that apply or can be applied to marketing efforts; these resources include money, time, people, and skills.

Microsoft® Project™ – A powerful planning and monitoring software tool used in developing plan schedules, assigning resources to tasks, and developing the plan budget.

MindManager™ – A software tool for brainstorming and planning by enabling planning teams within practices to design clear, well-planned documents at the beginning of the plan.

Mission – A statement that describes what the organization does, how it is done, and for whom it is done.

Monitoring – A procedure for checking the effectiveness and efficiency in implementing a plan by identifying its strengths and shortcomings and recommending corrective measures to optimize the intended outcomes.

Multispecialty group practices – Group practices that include multiple specialties and disciplines.

Network affiliations – The least-integrated type of alliance; functions as a club with a general purpose.

Objectives – Specific statements describing what the organization is trying to achieve.

Operational business plan – A plan that documents exactly how to operate the practice through items such as the detailed operating budget, detailed market and competitor research and analysis, product design specs, sales prospect lists, partner acquisition strategies, intellectual property strategy, and anything else that guides the growth of the venture.

Organization and analytical skills competency – A competency that demonstrates a systematic approach to problem solving, decision making, and the development and administration of systems to address day-to-day issues and the long-term improvement needs of the practice.

Organizational culture – The values, beliefs, and customs of an organization.

Performance risk – The probability that intended strategic goals of the alliance may not be achieved despite diligent cooperation among the partners.

Physician hospital organization (PHO) – An organization in which physicians and hospitals become partners in the delivery of health care.

Place – The means of having the product offering available to the target audience. Also known as distribution.

Planning – A formalized procedure to produce an articulated result, in the form of an integrated system of decisions.

Porter's Five Forces – A systematic and structured analysis of market structure and competitive situation.

Positioning – How the organization wants its services perceived by both customers and the competition.

Price – The value exchanged for the offering (e.g., service).

Product – What the actual offering (e.g., service) comprises.

Product mix – The set of all products and items that a particular seller offers for sale to buyers.

Professionalism Competency – A competency defined within the *ACMPE Guide to the Body of Knowledge for Medical Practice Management* that demonstrates a commitment to achieving professional standards that enhance personal and organizational integrity and contribute to the profession.

Program – A system of projects or services intended to meet a public need.

Promotion – The means of communicating the offering (e.g., service) to the target audience.

Relational risk – The probability that one or more partners do not comply with the rules governing the alliance.

Risk – Unanticipated variation or negative variation, which is typically associated with negative outcomes.

Service – The work done by one person or group that benefits another.

Service area – The geographic area and target market to be served by the practice.

Single-specialty group practices – Group practices that include only physicians of the same specialty and provide a significant level of integration.

Situational analysis – An in-depth process to develop understanding of the needs of specific audiences in a specific setting. It involves a combination of data-gathering techniques conducted from a variety of perspectives (social, economic, environmental, political, etc.).

Stakeholder – Any group or individual who can affect or who is affected by the achievement of a practice's objectives.

Stakeholder relationships – The relationships between the practice and its internal and external bodies of influence.

Start-up business plan – A plan used to convince potential investors to provide the practice with the necessary capital; sometimes referred to as an "idea" plan.

Strategic alliances – Alliances that allow two or more organizations to pool resources in order to gain access to up-to-date technology and maintain competitive advantage in hypercompetitive environments, such as health care.

Strategic planning – A disciplined effort to produce fundamental decisions and actions that shape and guide what an organization is, what it does, and why it does it, with a focus on the future.

Strategy – A systematic plan used to determine and reveal the organizational purpose in terms of long-term objectives, action programs, and resource allocation priorities.

SWOT analysis – An assessment of an organizations internal strengths and weaknesses and external opportunities and threats.

Target market – A specific group of consumers who have a want or need for the practice's services or products.

Technical/Professional Knowledge and Skills Competency – A competency defined within the *ACMPE Guide to the Body of Knowledge for Medical Practice Management* that demonstrates the knowledge and skills for job performance. It encompasses the knowledge, skills, behavior, beliefs, values, traits, and motives that drive superior performance.

Values – The core priorities in the organization's culture, including what members' priorities are and how they truly act in the organization.

Vision – A statement that describes a state that the organization is striving to achieve in the future.

About the Authors

Dawn M. Oetjen, PhD, MHA is a tenured associate professor and the director of the Graduate Program in Health Services Administration (HSA) at the University of Central Florida. She teaches courses at both the undergraduate and graduate levels. Dr. Oetjen has contributed to numerous peer-reviewed publications and regularly presents her research at academic and practitioner conferences, including presenting at MGMA's annual conferences in 2002, 2003, and 2004. In addition to her academic experience, Dr. Oetjen served as the Director of Quality Management, Case Management, Utilization Review, Health Information Management, and Support Services. She was also a Lister Hill Fellow at the Center for Quality Measurement and Improvement Agency for Health Care Policy and Research, U.S. Department of Health and Human Services, in Rockville, Maryland.

Reid M. Oetjen, PhD, MSHSA is a tenure-earning assistant professor and the assistant director of the Health Services Administration Programs at the University of North Florida. He teaches courses at both the undergraduate and graduate levels. Dr. Oetjen has contributed to numerous peer-reviewed publications and regularly presents his research at academic and practitioner conferences, including presenting at MGMA's annual conferences in 2002, 2003, and 2004. In addition to his academic experience, Dr. Oetjen served as the assistant administrator for a national skilled-nursing facility chain.

Index

Accounting,
  accrual, 42-43
  balance sheet, 43-45, 131
  cash-based, 43-46
  cash flow statement 44, 131
  discounted cash flow, 45
  equity, 45
  expenditures, 42-43
  income statement, 43-45,
    133
  return on investment, (ROI),
    19, 45
Advertising, 31, 42, 49, 55,
  58-60, 99
Alliances, 20, 75-79, 82-88,
  126-128, 136-137
American College of Medical
  Practice Executives,
  (ACMPE), v, 9-11, 111,
  137, 139
American Marketing
  Association, (AMA), 54,
  125
Analysis,
  consumer, 51-52, 132
  internal practice, 51
  macroenvironmental, 51, 134
  market, 40-42, 51-52, 55,
    134, 137
  microenvironmental, 135
  Porter's Five Forces , 52-53
  situational, 50-52, 138
  skills, 9, 11, 15, 136
Assets, 37, 39, 44-45, 80-81,
  131-134
Awareness building, 94

Balanced scorecard, 69-70, 131
Bank-financing plan, 37-39,
  131
Baseline indicators, 106-108,
  130
Bedside manner, 106-108, 130
Benchmark, 40, 69, 97, 131
Break-even worksheet, 43-44
Business Plan,
  components, 40

financial, 42-45
executive summary, 41-42
getting started, 39
monitoring, 63-73
management, 46-47
operational, 37-38
reporting, 70-72
risk tolerance, 46
start-up, 37-39, 138
systems design, 69

Cash flow statement, 44
Certified Medical Practice
  Executive, (CMPE), vii, 5-6
Community
  collaboration, 94-95
  focus, 94
  involvement, 95
  outreach, 21, 91-97
Communications skills, 9-10,
  15, 132
Competitive
  advantage, 51-54
  pricing, 57, 76
  rivalry, 53-54
  strategy, 79, 125
Conflict, 77, 85, 88
Consumer analysis, 50-54, 132
Conventional planning, 24
Corporation, 41, 87-88, 121,
  128
Cost-plus pricing, 57, 132
Cultural
  humility, 128
  sensitivity, 95
Culture of customer service,
  105-106, 129
Current assets and liabilities, 45
Customer
  difficult, 107
  relations programs, 21, 91,
    108
  service, 105-108

Data collecting, 96
Demand pricing, 57